FLORIDA

DogOwner's

HANDBOOK

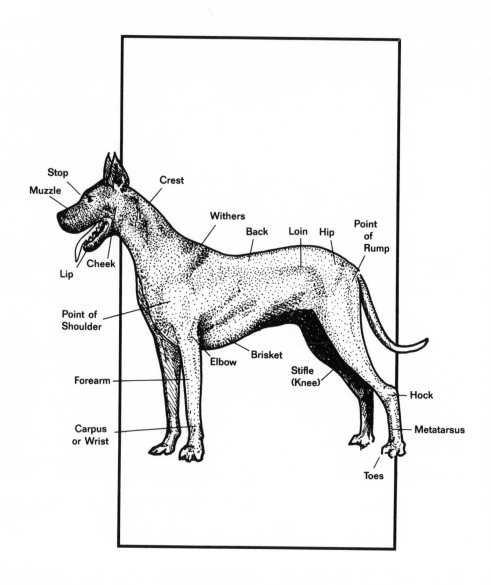

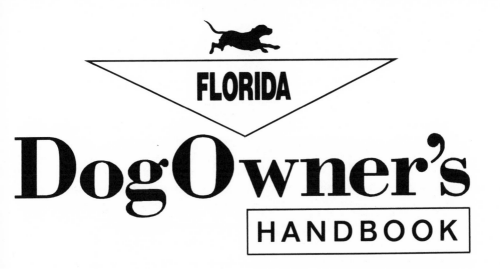

FLORIDA
DogOwner's
HANDBOOK

Marty Marth

Pineapple Press
Sarasota, Florida

Inquiries should be addressed to
Pineapple Press, Inc., P.O. Drawer 16008, Southside Station, Sarasota, Florida 34239.

Library of Congress Cataloging-in-Publication Data

Marth, Marty
    Florida dog owner's handbook / by Marty Marth. — 1st ed.
        p.   cm.
    ISBN 0-910923-72-8 : $12.95 (est.)
    1. Dogs—Florida. 2. Dogs—Diseases—Florida. I. Title.
SF427.M36   1990
636.7'009759—dc20   89-49067
                                                                          CIP

First edition

10 9 8 7 6 5 4 3 2 1

Design by Joan Lange Kresek
Composition by E. T. Lowe, Nashville, Tennessee

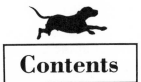

Contents

ACKNOWLEDGMENTS

The author would like to thank Dr. Donald Wolfersteig, DVM, whose tactful suggestions vastly improved this work. He and his veterinary colleagues throughout the state perform daily miracles keeping our beloved dogs alive and well.

Appreciation goes also to veterinary assistants Melissa Ware and Mimi Kessler, who cheerfully helped with technical information and addresses needed by the author.

And finally, a tip of the author's hat to Ms. Lee Burnham of the Alachua County Humane Society, whose love of animals is surpassed only by her steadfast pursuit of anyone who abuses them.

> **"** *DOG: A kind of subsidiary Deity designed to catch the surplus of the world's worship.*
> *—Ambrose Bierce* **"**

Introduction

F lorida is a relatively young state, mostly unsettled until after 1845 when it was admitted to the Union. Even its animal life documented by fossils reveals a late-blooming land that emerged from the sea about 50 million years ago, after the Age of Dinosaurs had passed. The state's fossil digs also yield remains of canines—ferocious hyenas, wolves, and coyotes—that roamed Florida about five million years ago.

As far as scientists can tell, humans did not arrive on the Florida peninsula until a mere 10,000 years ago. And while no written records attest to just when a Floridian first domesticated a dog, the evidence indicates there were as many dogs around the campfire centuries ago as there were Timucuan or Calusa Indians.

Early white settlers showed a similar appreciation for the dog. Works of art from the past five centuries of rule by Spaniards, Frenchmen, and Britishers—a succession of gold-lusting explorers, bloodthirsty pirates, soul-seeking missionaries, and Indian-hunting soldiers—show them cutting their way through the state's hinterlands in the company of tail-wagging dogs.

And some things never change, at least in Florida. As they have for centuries, people are still coming to the Sunshine State. The immigrants aren't called explorers anymore, but tourists, an estimated 38 million a year. A record 50,000 of them stay on each year to become new residents. For some, Florida is a shady spot with a cold drink on a pearl-white beach, or the healing balm of a warm sun on an arthritic shoulder. For others, it's a fresh start with a young family and a new job in a booming city. Whatever the reason, many arrive in Florida with a dog. Others, perhaps anticipating spending more time outdoors or longing for companionship in a new home, obtain a dog when they get here.

Statistics compiled by the Pet Food Institute in Washington, D.C., reveal that one of every five persons in the nation owns a dog. Presuming Florida's dog-owning population follows the national trend, that comes to 2.6 million Floridian canines. In economic terms, the numbers are just as staggering. Americans spend $13 billion a year on the feed and care of their pets, be they dogs, cats, horses, exotic pets, or birds. That figure includes such luxury items as dog collars, rawhide chews, and after-bath colognes. As best as can be determined, Florida dog owners' share of that ever-increasing expenditure comes to around $139 million.

Dog-owning tastes in the Sunshine State differ little from national trends as far as pet food choices and monies spent on veterinary bills go. But that may be where the similarities in dog care end. For as many transplants soon learn, Florida demands a new lifestyle. The state's heat, humidity, and insects quickly reshape how an owner cares for Fido. And no newcomer has been prepared for the harrowing scene of an inattentive pup being chased by an alligator.

"We never had a problem with this back home" is a familiar refrain in any Florida veterinarian's office. To which, of course, the animal doctor stifles a response such as, "Well, you've got a problem with it now!"

This book is designed to benefit those new Floridians as well as long-time and native-born residents by helping make life in Florida as enjoyable and problem-free for their dogs as it is for them.

❝I had a little dog and
my dog was very small,
He licked me in the face,
and he answered to my call.
Of all the treasures
that were mine
I loved him most of all.
* —Frances Cornford❞*

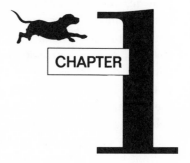

CHAPTER

1

A Place in the Sun

A vast array of canines call Florida home. Classified advertisements sell wolf hybrids, while in the territory around the Suwannee River, coyotes roam at will. As for domesticated dogs, every breed can be found in the state, although where in the state the various breeds are likely to be found says much about the character of Florida's different regions.

For example, Miami Beach apartment or condominium dwellers are more apt to keep toy poodles and other such small breeds. Toward the rural reaches of the state, as undeveloped acreage increases, so does the size of the resident dogs. Sporting breeds such as retrievers, working breeds such as Rottweilers, and the hound breeds are more commonly found where population density shrinks.

WHY HAVE A PET DOG?

An obvious reason to own a dog is the companionship that it provides. This long-known comradeship has spawned a new branch of human behavioral study, dubbed "petology" by some. It researches the profound effect pets can have on people.

For children, a dog can be an invaluable friend. It is a buddy that provides not only entertainment and companionship but can teach responsibility. Experts say that for children and teens, pets also add stability to a household. They point out that as the young person's life changes, or when grandparents die, or the household moves, or a parental divorce occurs, or human friends come and go, or schools change, often it is the family pet that remains the same. "The dog is the old family friend in a changing world, the one that helps people get through the rough spots," says one petologist. The family pet also serves as an emotional outlet, lending an uncritical ear to the 99 percent of dog owners whom studies report talk to Rover.

Young working couples, especially those who do not yet have children, may inadvertently use the dog as a surrogate child, which helps the couple function as a "real family" and gives the couple a chance to learn and to accept responsibility for an additional family member. This presence of a dog in the household, say the behaviorists, may make the couple's transition into parenthood easier.

Similarly, in the elderly person's life a dog becomes a vital member of the family, a best friend that actually can make a health difference. University studies of heart attack patients reveal that patients who own dogs (and other pets) are more likely to recuperate following medical treatment. One such study at the University of Maryland showed that stroking and talking to a dog consistently lowers blood pressure and gives people a sense of well-being. In 1982, the American Veterinary Medical Association officially recognized these studies and established the Committee on the Human-Animal Bond to investigate further how pets affect human health. It is a field that behaviorists describe as "a new frontier."

Research indicates that a dog in the household of elderly persons may provide still other benefits, such as:

—forcing the person to exercise and socialize by taking the dog for walks (a London study found that persons tend to be more sociable while walking their dog than when they walk without the dog);

—giving a focus to the life of a person who may live alone by keeping the owner busy and entertained;

—prompting an elderly person to maintain good health because of the responsibility of caring for the dog;

—adding a sense of security by protecting the household and barking at strangers who come to the door.

DOG OWNERSHIP IN FLORIDA

There are few "musts" in the selection of a dog that can live comfortably in Florida, but rare is the Sunshine State veterinarian who will recommend heavily furred, traditionally cold-climate breeds such as the Chow Chow or Siberian husky. These breeds simply are uncomfortable in Florida's heat and humidity and often have difficulty acclimating.

In fact, the state's hot and humid climate is regarded by some dog enthusiasts with downright trepidation. The famous Morristown, New Jersey, guide-dog training company, The Seeing Eye, Inc., avoids putting training sites in Florida. "Our own experience taught us that the sunny South was not the best place to train Seeing Eye dogs," its public information spokesperson explained. The spokesperson pointed out that the business of training dogs for the blind began in Nashville, Tennessee, in 1929, but even that locale proved too warm. A company official reported, "The dogs did not hold up well for summer training, so we moved north to New Jersey where the climate was cooler and more varied, and where the dogs not only worked harder but suffered less often from skin ailments."

Another of the musts regarding dog ownership in Florida is the law that regulates buying and selling puppies. It prohibits the sale of any puppy less than eight weeks old. In addition, any dog that is sold must have a health certificate, must have received vaccinations, and must be free of external and internal parasites.

In addition to that state requirement, some counties in Florida have their own local ordinances that affect dog ownership and care. Miami's Dade County, for example, passed a hotly contested ordinance in April 1989 designed to prevent an increase in the number of pit bulldogs that reside in that county. The ordinance, which has survived one court challenge, prevents newcomers from bringing their pit bulldogs into the county, and it imposes strict guidelines on Dade residents who already own them. Residents must register their pit bulls, keep them securely confined, carry either $300,000 liability insurance or show "other financial liability," and must not walk their dogs within fifty feet of any public school.

In Alachua County, where the University of Florida is situated, all dogs and cats must wear rabies vaccination tags at all times. Alachua's neighboring counties have no such ordinance.

Counties in Florida, at the local health department's edict, may completely restrict the movement of a dog. Alachua County, for example, imposed a temporary, total quarantine on its canine residents during the summer of 1989 because of a rabies outbreak and confiscated any dogs found to be running loose.

So laws, permanent and temporary, concerning Florida dogs will vary (see Chapter 14 for more legal information). But nearly all major Florida cities have leash laws. It is a good idea for newcomers to check with their local humane society or animal shelter officials to find out what, if any, requirements exist in a particular area. In addition, persons who live in apartments, condominiums, or mobile home parks should check their rental agreement or declaration of condominium or bylaws to make sure pets are allowed.

WHERE TO OBTAIN A DOG

The fundamental decision that confronts a prospective dog purchaser is not which puppy to buy but whether to buy from a pet store or from a breeder. It would seem not to matter as long the pup is healthy, but an increasing number of veterinarians discourage their customers from purchasing dogs from any source but reputable breeders.

Pet stores abound in Florida, the nation's fourth most populous state, and many engage in the profitable business of offering a wide variety of dogs for sale. The state is also not without its disreputable breeders. Veterinarians' recommendations to purchase a dog only from a reputable breeder are not intended to indict all pet stores but only those stores that purchase their supply of puppies from so-called puppy mills. Many such mills are inhumane breeding factories where newborns are kept in limited, and often filthy, confines.

Prior to 1981, puppies from these mills arrived in the state without inoculation for any diseases. As a result, some dogs died during shipment and others arrived in Florida half dead or generally unhealthy. These conditions prompted the state to pass a strict law in 1981 requiring that incoming dogs (or dogs born in Florida) be vaccinated for distemper, hepatitis, leptospirosis, tracheobronchitis (kennel cough), and canine parvovirus.

Not only were puppies arriving from suppliers in poor health, but they also carried potential future problems such as hip dysplasia or other genetically produced ailments. This still occurs when a disreputable breeder or a puppy mill does not maintain good breeding practices and permits dogs carrying "bad" genes to continue reproducing. Another problem with dogs bred by unsavory breeders or puppy mills is that many of the pups are never handled by humans until they are shipped out for sale.

Thus, a reputable breeding kennel is usually a safer place from

There are more than 2,000 practicing veterinarians in Florida. Not all treat small animals such as dogs, but here are a few tips for dog owners, especially first-timers, seeking a good veterinarian:

—Call your local animal shelter or humane society for some veterinarians' names.

—Ask friends who are happy with their veterinarian for a recommendation.

—Select a veterinarian who is conveniently located and then schedule a visit. Ask about his or her attitudes toward pet care. Check fees, and compare. Always inquire as to whether there are extra costs for emergency or after-hours calls. Observe, too, whether the office is clean and professional.

which to buy puppies. The reasoning is that, first, the breeder takes pride in the litters produced by his or her kennel—bright, healthy, well-conformed pups are the breeder's best advertisement. For once the word spreads that a certain kennel produces genetically deficient pups, it is certain public relations death. And second, a breeder most often intends to stay in business at the same location for a long time. Unhappy dog owners know where to return the dog. In the case of pet stores, which may accept returns (though not always), the seller can only offer the excuse that the puppy came from out of state.

So if you fall in love with a pet store pup and must have it, do some homework. Find out how long the store has been in business and whether it has had any complaints against it from the area humane society. Talk to the manager and the staff to see how knowledgeable they are about dogs, breeds, and diseases. Ask what the guarantee is on the pup against its exhibiting a disease once you have taken it home. A reputable pet store will gladly discuss these matters and offer to take the pup back, within a reasonable period of time, if it is not healthy.

Another source of puppies is the local humane society, or what once was called simply "the pound." In recent years, city and county officials have opted to shed the old "pound" image for the kindlier "shelter." By any name, it is a holding facility for hundreds of lost or abandoned animals, most of which end up being destroyed.

Everyone has heard stories about the dog who was rescued from a shelter and went on to become a canine movie star. Most of these are indeed stories and may be the figment of some publicist's imagination. That's not to say that a good dog cannot be found in animal shelters. Anyone who has ever visited such facilities finds the experience heart-breaking as every little button-nosed mongrel wags and pleads to be taken home.

Occasionally, a selective shelter customer can find a marvelous purebred dog. But caution should be used. There may be a sound reason why a sleek Doberman or sturdy dachshund is at the shelter—and it is not because the dog was "lost." It may be generally bad tempered. Or perhaps it snaps at children. It may be sickly. Keep in mind that by the time most dogs reach an animal shelter, they are mature or nearly so. The previous owner may have learned at the last veterinary checkup that the dog is developing a health problem. In a few instances, the purebred dog is a "cull," unwanted by its breeders because it does not meet specifications, although most responsible breeders dispose of their culls. Fortunately, shelters generally require the spaying or neutering of adopted dogs so the culls will not (and should not) be used for breeding.

The real animal shelter treasures often turn out to be the mutts. Any prospective dog owner who simply wants a companion dog is well advised to select a mixed-breed dog from a shelter. Not only is there a good chance that a nice pet is about to join the family, but the owner has a good feeling about saving one dog from a near-certain death sentence. More importantly, mutts seem to do well in Florida's subtropical climate, being hardy enough to shake off some of the sophisticated diseases, not to mention an influx of fleas, that might disable the more fashionable but less tolerant purebred.

SELECTING A DOG

How does anybody know whether a certain dog is the right one? One way is to devise a mental "résumé" that the canine "applicant" must fit.

First, where the dog will live should be considered. Larger breeds such as the retrievers, setters, Rottweilers, Great Danes, and boxers are more suited to the great outdoors with plenty of running room. That can be hard to find in many of Florida's metropolitan areas. The toy breeds as well as small spaniels, hounds, and terriers can live in a home or apartment quite nicely.

The next consideration should be the family's configuration. If there are small children in the household, some thought should be

Parents seeking a first pet for children would do well to adopt an adult dog. It may take more time to find just the perfect pet, but adult dogs are less likely to be overly rowdy with a young child who may be timid around animals. Adult dogs also may arrive with bonus talents, having already been housebroken, obedience trained, and taught some tricks. Local humane societies or animal shelters offer many such canine gems.

given to the dog's temperament. Some breeds such as the retrievers and setters tend to be more forgiving if a small child pulls the dog's ear or tail. Even puppies can snap at people, and such behavior can foretell an adult dog that is going to be short on patience.

Once the size and breed of dog are selected, it's time for Fido's résumé to be more specific. The owner should know how the puppy has been reared. Most dog experts believe that from birth to two weeks of age, the puppy must have a close association with its mother. If this has not occurred, a puppy may have been malnourished. At about three weeks, the puppy is developing its motor skills and begins to explore its environment. The most critical time is next, as the puppy learns to get along with its brothers and sisters. This occurs from about four weeks to fourteen weeks. Human contact is important during this time for the pup to learn to accept being handled by people.

Every litter produces pups with different personalities ranging from aggressive to timid. Most experts recommend selecting the most alert and curious pup. These characteristics generally reflect an animal that is intelligent and healthy. A timid pup may not feel well or may not have been handled enough.

Puppies also come in different sizes ranging from Rambo to runt. Most dog experts recommend one of the mid-sized models because they generally mature to be better examples of the breed. Other traits to seek are relatively straight legs (few puppies are perfect) and a well-proportioned body, despite the fact that a puppy's feet and bones may seem oddly oversized. The dog's teeth should look even and should close properly with the upper front teeth closing neatly over the lower teeth.

Prospective dog buyers should also never assume that because a pup is the progeny of champion parents it is a junior champion awaiting its day in the show ring. Reputable breeders admit that it is difficult to determine whether an eight-week-old pup is a future trophy winner. Purchasers should be wary of any seller who "guarantees" that a small puppy is a "sure winner." In truth, breeders concede that even the most auspiciously bred puppy has only a one-in-seven chance of ever seeing a blue ribbon.

Avoid a pup four months old or older that has not been previously handled. By this age, a dog may have developed what is called "kennel dog syndrome." Such dogs know only their kennel home—often a small crate—and may never satisfactorily adapt to humans. Kennel syndrome dogs are pitiful, really. And while otherwise shy, they often exhibit aggressive behavior such as biting—not out of viciousness but out of fear. Expert handlers report a complete cure of these misbehaviors once the kennel syndrome dogs are returned to their original environments.

Not all the responsibility of dog ownership rests with the dog's behavior. Another aspect of the dog résumé rests with the owner. Dogs are not playthings. And some owners clearly do not deserve their faithful canine buddies.

Owners must be willing to take their dogs, puppies particularly, outside in the Florida heat for walks. The alternative is paper training. Puppies under twelve weeks old usually cannot "hold it" longer than two hours. That means a lot of newspapers or a lot of trips outdoors for the owner. Once housebroken, dogs still require exercise. Outings should be made several times a day.

Another responsibility is the regular veterinary care that dogs require. Vaccinations and deworming should be given at regular intervals, and unless it is intended as a breeding animal, the pup should be spayed or neutered once it reaches six months of age.

The list goes on. No dog is pleasant to live with unless it has manners and will, at least minimally, obey its owner. Many owners believe that it is cruel to demand that a dog come when it is called or sit on command. It is not cruel. In fact, such obedience training can save the dog's life.

Nearly every Florida city or county has an obedience training school. Fees are reasonable, well worth the results that are often achieved. These schools can be fun or drudgery, depending on what the owner makes it. Although the occasional blockheaded pup comes along, most dogs can actually enjoy training sessions. As for the owner, the rewards of having an obedient dog will last a lifetime. Owners who prefer large dog breeds such as German shepherds, Doberman pinschers, Great Danes, or Rottweilers soon may find that obedience school is their best ally. It's no fun to be taken for an evening run by a 125-pound dog.

The secret to training a dog is to know when your dog is ready to learn. Many authorities recommend that training begin at about eight weeks. But some breeds mature more slowly and may need to begin lessons at three months. The dog, believe it or not, will indicate its readiness by responding enthusiastically to the work and its owner's rewarding praise and a treat. Adult dogs also benefit from obedience training, but results may not occur as quickly or as thoroughly as with a pup.

By now, it must be obvious that responsible dog ownership can be time consuming. For that reason, persons who work full-time, or put in many overtime hours, may have difficulty providing the attention that a dog demands. Any dog, but especially a puppy, that is left to fend for itself for hours on end in a house or apartment is certain to work mischief. Much of that troublemaking can be serious and can cost the dog owner a security deposit. Soiled carpeting, torn or eaten wallpaper, and shredded draperies can land the renter out on the sidewalk with pooch in hand.

SPAYING AND NEUTERING

Most experts agree that neutered or spayed dogs make better pets for a variety of reasons:

—Male dogs are less apt to mark territory with aromatic bodily discharges.

—The dog may be a more affectionate pet, unhindered by bodily cycles and passionate distractions.

—Male dogs will stray less, making them more unlikely to encounter contagious diseases or death by poisoning, automobiles, or gunshots.

—Female dogs will keep their surroundings cleaner when they are free of the estrous reproductive cycle.

—Male dogs will be less likely to contract prostatic disease. Female dogs will less often contract uterine disorders.

—There will be no unwanted puppies that the owner must either find homes for or have destroyed.

—Female dogs that are spayed prior to their second estrus will have a greatly reduced chance of mammary cancer later in life.

Unless a dog is a well-pedigreed, well-conformed, show-quality animal, there is little reason to bring more puppies into the world. Thousands of perfectly healthy and adorable but unwanted canines are carted to Florida's humane societies and animal shelters each week. The vast majority are put to death. The cost of picking up strays and caring for abandoned, abused, or unwanted dogs soars each year, and taxpayers shell out millions of dollars to maintain these services. Experts agree that spaying female dogs and neutering males is the most inexpensive and humane solution to this overpopulation problem.

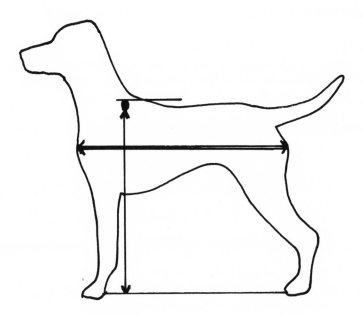

A dog's height is measured from the ground to the top of the shoulder. Length measuring is from the point of the shoulder to the point of the hindquarters.

> *Fox terriers are born with about four times as much original sin in them as other dogs.*
> —*Jerome K. Jerome*

CHAPTER

2

A Bevy of Breeds

From a few wild species, notably wolves, jackals, and dingo-type canines, more than 400 modern dog breeds have evolved over the past thousands of years. Some developed naturally, adapting to various global climates and food sources. Breeds in cold climates grew dense, almost oily, fur coats. Warm-climate breeds developed short, sometimes barely noticeable coats. Coat colors also evolved to permit dogs to blend with their environment and stalk prey more successfully. Survivors passed the best traits on to their descendants.

Obtaining food also was more successful when dogs hunted in packs. Pack hunting often was necessary because few canines have great speed, but most do have tremendous endurance. In packs, dogs could track prey until the victim tired and the pack could close in for the kill.

Some canines were selectively cultivated by humans who preferred certain traits above others, although the specific wild stock from which these domestic dogs were bred remains unknown. Herdsmen, for example, developed canines that displayed an instinct for keeping herds or flocks of animals moving and safe from predators. Such training must have taken time, for the herding dog first had to be convinced not to attack the herd members. Hunters, on the other hand, tended toward dogs that could track or retrieve game. Middle Eastern alabaster relief panels dating back to 668 B.C. depict mastiffs, collared and leashed, being led by men to hunt lions. Still other types or breeds were used by Native Americans as camp guards and to pull travois.

Among people with increasing leisure time has come a demand for what could be termed "luxury" dog breeds—dogs that have their roots in the predawn world of hunting but that have been bred to the easy life as companion animals. Many of today's dog owners prefer cute and cuddly models such as the shih tzu, Lhasa apso, toy poodle, and Yorkshire terrier because they fit nicely into apartment or condominium lifestyles.

The notion of pigeonholing dog breeds into specific types began with dog shows. Such shows originated in England, where, as a wag once remarked, "Put any two Britishers together and they'll make a contest out of something." The first English dog show was in 1859; eleven years later Americans imported the event.

When the twentieth century began, so-called fixed or purebreeds emerged. A purebred dog breeds true and reveals consistent traits of color and conformation. Such traits have become breed standards that show-quality purebred dogs must meet.

In 1884 the American Kennel Club was formed, and it remains the last word in purebred canine pedigree throughout much of the Western

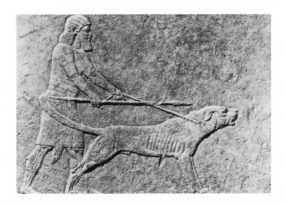

This bas relief dated about 630 B.C. from the ancient city of Nineveh depicts lion hunters using mastiff type dogs. (British Museum, London)

Hemisphere. Today the AKC recognizes approximately 125 dog breeds. Such official recognition is achieved once the AKC opens a studbook for that breed. There are seven classifications: sporting dogs, working dogs, hounds, terriers, toy breeds, herding breeds, and nonsporting dogs. Some AKC-recognized shows also include an "unclassified" grouping for dog breeds that have not been in existence long enough to prove they breed to a consistent standard.

Heights and weights in the following descriptions are approximate to give readers an idea of the size of each of these breeds. The lesser height or weight indicates the average female's size, while the greater height and weight is that of an average male dog.

SPORTING BREEDS

These breeds tend to include large dogs that are known for their generally easygoing temperament. Sporting breeds scent their prey, usually birds, through the air. Breeders of these dogs have been cautious to maintain the physical stamina for which these animals are prized. Sporting dogs include the retrievers, spaniels, setters, pointers, griffons, and Weimaraners.

Retrievers, be they golden, Labrador, Chesapeake Bay, flat-coated or curly-coated, generally weigh in at 50 pounds or better. They earned their name because they have been bred to retrieve prey and carry it to the hunter. Exuberance and a love of the outdoors make them ideal canine companions of hikers, hunters, and boaters. These breeds usually love the water and are excellent swimmers.

Golden retrievers possess a dense, medium-long coat in several varieties of golden color. They are sturdily built and display a smooth, free gait when they move. This breed came into popular use in England and Scotland in the early 1800s. They stand from 21 to 24 inches at the shoulder and weigh from 60 to 70 pounds.

Labrador retrievers, like their golden cousins, are sturdy, active dogs. Their coats are black, yellow, or chocolate-colored, are short and dense, and feel somewhat stiff. Despite the "Labrador" label, the breed originated in Newfoundland, from where enthusiasts imported the breed to England in the 1830s. Trademarks of this breed include its marvelous disposition and a tail that resembles that of an otter.

Chesapeake Bay retriever breeders boast that theirs is an especially hardy animal, able to withstand extremely cold weather. Its general build is very similar to that of the other retrievers, but its color varies more, from a dark brown to a tan color. The size range of this most affable breed is from 21 to 26 inches at the shoulder and 55 to 80 pounds.

Anyone purchasing a retriever for use as a hunting dog should select an animal that displays no hesitancy about entering water. Retrievers do well in Florida, although some individuals tend to gain weight easily and the weight can be cumbersome outdoors in the state's heat and humidity. For that reason, retrievers must be regularly exercised and their diets monitored.

Like their retrieving cousins, spaniels come in a variety of types, including Brittany, cocker, springer, field, Clumber, and Sussex. Sporting dogs that they are, they enjoy a good romp in the woods and are adept at swimming. With their mild dispositions, they generally are excellent with children.

Most spaniels have medium to long coats, which does not seem to cause them much of a problem in Florida's subtropical climate, although if left outdoors spaniels tend to dig a napping hole in which to cool off.

Brittany spaniels weigh 30 to 40 pounds and stand about 19 inches at the shoulder. They are extremely popular hunting dogs, possibly because they are the only spaniels that will point toward quarry. The breed is naturally tail-less, and its coloring is orange or liver-colored, and white.

Cocker spaniels are among the smallest, most popular, and best known of the sporting breeds. Height is from 14 to 15 inches at the shoulder, and weight is about 25 pounds. Cockers are delightful pets whose coats, of any color, may be straight or wavy. The fur is long but is frequently clipped, a plus in Florida's heat and humidity. The origin of the cocker's name derives from the dog's skill in hunting woodcock.

English springer spaniels, 19 inches at the shoulder and weighing 49 to 55 pounds, were developed in England as field dogs. They not only flush game from the woodlands and fields but retrieve as well. An English springer's coat generally is medium long, feathery, flat or wavy, and is either white with liver-red, liver and white with tan, or roan colors of either blue or liver.

Setters first earned their name because they were expected to crouch before prey. Nowadays, however, they are more aptly termed pointers. The **Irish setter** is often considered the glamorous sporting dog, and few dog lovers have not been struck by the beauty of its gleaming bronze coat. Some dog experts, however, allege that the "brains have been bred out" of some setters so that today's specimens tend to be hyperactive and goofy. But given enough room to romp, they settle down, and their marvelous disposition makes them ideal family pets. The Irish setter, developed in the 1700s in Ireland as a field hunter, stands 25 to 27 inches at the shoulder and may weigh between 60 and 70 pounds. The colors of these beauties in the U.S. generally range from liver-red to orange-bronze. In their Irish homeland, more white markings adorn the breed.

English setters stand about 25 inches at the shoulder and weigh 60 pounds. They are lovely animals with long, silken coats and date back in England to the 1500s. They come in a variety of colors, ranging from pure white to mixtures of yellow, liver, orange, and blue or black with white. Overall flecks of color are preferred by enthusiasts to large, solid spots.

Gordon setters gained their name because they were popular with Scotland's fourth duke of Gordon in the late 1700s. Known for an eagerness to work, they are faithful companions and family dogs for owners who can provide adequate exercise space. Gordons measure from 23 to 27 inches at the shoulder and weigh from 45 to 80 pounds. A typically lovely Gordon setter coat is properly shiny black with tan markings, and may be wavy or straight.

As their name suggests, the pointers in the sporting dog group direct hunters to prey by freezing rigidly in place, pointing with their bodies to the quarry. Evidently, the predisposition to point is a highly dominant trait because dogs lacking obvious pointer breed standards can exhibit this behavior. Because pointers also retrieve, this sporting breed is considered by some to be more versatile than retrievers or setters.

The **German shorthaired pointer** has many advantages. Good-natured, intelligent, excellent with children, and a superb hunting companion, this breed also affords easy care. The breed's coat is short, close-lying, and requires virtually no grooming. The German shorthaired pointer is happiest, however, with some running room to exercise its sturdy frame. This breed stands about two feet at the shoulder and weighs about 65 pounds.

German wirehaired pointers developed in their namesake country in the late 1800s and were not seen with any frequency in the United States until the 1920s. They stand about two feet tall at the shoulder and weigh 60 pounds. As their name suggests, their coats, usually liver-red and white, are bristly stiff and cover a dense undercoat that generally thins out in the summertime.

Wirehaired pointing griffons originated in Holland and were adapted for hunting in swampy regions. They are distinguished by a long head and a gray-tinged, wiry coat that features splotches of chestnut markings. The breed stands about 20 inches tall.

Among the aristocrats of the sporting group is the **Weimaraner**. Large, well-muscled, and nicely proportioned, these dogs are highly prized for their intelligence and beauty. Shoulder height is between 23 and 27 inches and this breed weighs from 55 to 85 pounds. The state's hot, moist climate does not severely affect this breed because its coat is naturally short. Coloring of this breed is an outstanding feature, as most are a misty, almost metallic-looking gray. Its eyes are amber, gray, or blue-gray. The breed was perfected as a bird dog in Germany in the 1800s.

WORKING BREEDS

Breeds in this class were originally developed, as their name implies, to work. Humans have extensively used these breeds, some of which are among the dog world's largest and strongest. From Siberian huskies to Great Danes, this grouping comprises the most breeds.

While the majority of working dog breeds make loving pets, owners should realize that these animals often exhibit a "bred-for-work" mentality. As a result, while many enjoy frolicking with the family, they are happiest when working at such tasks as guarding the family home. They sometimes tend to exhibit a businesslike temperament, occasionally lacking patience with children. Most dog experts recommend that working dog breeds be given some obedience training. Besides, these canine workaholics generally relish being put through their classroom paces.

Alaskan malamutes are sturdy and strong. Although only two feet high at the shoulder, a male malamute can weigh up to 85 pounds, much of it pure muscle. Raised for centuries as a sled dog (though it is improper to call this breed a "husky"), the malamute is a cold-weather canine with a coat to match. The coat is a dense, furry covering of gray or black with white markings underlain by a woolly mat of hair. Few veterinarians recommend Florida as the ideal home for Alaskan malamutes. These dogs simply are too uncomfortable in the heat and humidity. If kept in air conditioning or thoroughly clipped, however, some of these dogs fare satisfactorily.

Boxers are protective of the home and family while patient with children. They generally stand 21 to 25 inches at the shoulder and weigh from 60 to 75 pounds. This breed is happy in Florida. Its smooth, flat-lying coat can be brindle, brown, or fawn with or without white markings. Boxers originally were bred in Europe for fighting

Experts caution that careless breeding of slim-hipped, large chested breeds such as Rottweilers is resulting in an increase of whelping problems, and veterinarians are performing more caesarean sections to deliver their pups safely.

and have been used in Germany as police dogs. They are often wary of strangers and take their yard-guarding duties seriously.

Doberman pinschers, long categorized as fierce guard or police dogs, are gracefully sleek animals named for Louis Doberman, a German who developed the breed in the late 1800s. "Dobies," as they are affectionately called, possess a strength that their agile frame belies. Doberman pinschers stand 24–28 inches at the shoulder and weigh 65–70 pounds. Their sleek, short coats are black, reddish-brown, blue, or a lesser-seen fawn. Rusty-tan markings always adorn the solid coloring. Because of their fierce reputation, partly due to cinematic portrayals, Dobermans in recent years are being bred to enhance their gentle dispositions. This breed is intelligent, keen to please, and makes a devoted pet.

Great Danes were developed in Germany from the mastiff breed more than 400 years ago to hunt wild boar. The Great Dane is a bold, elegant dog that is also one of the largest of breeds. A typical Dane can measure up to 30 inches at the shoulder and weigh up to 150 pounds. Its short, close coat is seen in colors of brindle, fawn, steel-blue, black, and the spotted harlequin. Because of its sheer size, obedience training a Great Dane is important. It also is critical that such a large animal be given sufficient living space and exercise. Despite its size, this breed is affectionate and generally patient with children or other pets.

Rottweilers, like Great Danes, descended from mastiff stock brought to Germany before 300 A.D. by the Romans. German locals in the vicinity of Rottweil prized this strong, intelligent breed and used it for moving and guarding livestock and for pulling sleds and carts. The Rottweiler's shorthaired coat is black with well-defined rusty-tan markings. A hallmark of this breed is its robust build, about 22 to 27 inches at the shoulder and 75 to more than 100 pounds of weight. Because of the strength of "Rotties," owners should ensure that the dog understands obedience rules and gets sufficient exercise. This breed is a bona fide working dog and may grow annoyed with teasing. For this reason, specialty Rottweiler guidebooks recommend that children not be left unattended with this breed.

Heavily furred **St. Bernards** sometimes find Florida summers uncomfortably long. These mountain dogs were traditionally used in the cold of the Swiss Alps and take their name from the St. Bernard Pass, where monks used the dogs to rescue snow travelers. The breed has been credited with saving the lives of some 2,000 humans. A St. Bernard measures about 26 to 29 inches at the shoulder and weighs a sturdy 140 to 170 pounds. There are shorthaired versions of this breed. Standard coat colors are white, red, or brindle.

Samoyeds, classified by dog references as an Arctic breed, feature a glorious double coat of weather-resistant fur that ranges from white to a cream color. This breed is thought to have originated in frigid northern Siberia thousands of years ago, where it was used as a reindeer herder and draft animal. Samoyeds are strong for their size, which generally is about 19 to 23 inches at the shoulder. They weigh between 35 and 65 pounds. Their name is a derivation of the Russian word *Samoed*, which is the name of groups of people who live in the Arkhangelsk region of the USSR. This is another of the cold-weather breeds that find the heat and humidity of Florida a sometimes insurmountable health obstacle, so care should be used before importing one of these dogs from colder climes.

Schnauzers come in three sizes, thus a version to suit just about everybody. Only two of the three sizes, the giant and standard schnauzers, are considered working dogs; the miniature version is classified as a terrier. This jaunty breed had its beginning in Germany. The giant schnauzer, dating back to the 1800s, ranges in height from 23 to 27 inches and weighs between 65 and 78 pounds. The standard schnauzer, recorded in Germany as far back as the 1400s, is slightly smaller and lighter, between 17 and 20 inches at the shoulder with a weight of 27 to 37 pounds. (The miniature schnauzer is discussed in the "Terriers" section.) Schnauzers are wirehaired dogs whose coloring may be black or silver or a combination of both. Clipped, these dogs have eyebrows, a mustache, and beard, which tends to give their faces a great deal of personality. They are agile and graceful and make good Florida pets if kept clipped.

Siberian huskies are the essence of the Arctic sled dog and are the only Arctic dog that is correctly termed a "husky." Robust and durable, these dogs generally stand about 20 to 24 inches at the shoulder and weigh 35 to 60 pounds. Their coats are virtually weather resistant, and colors are usually black, white, gray, or tan. Like the

Samoyed, the Siberian husky dates back thousands of years to the wintry cold of Siberia. It is not a breed that often gets the "thumbs up" from Florida veterinarians because its heavy coat and exercise demands can prompt health problems in the Sunshine State. In spite of its strength, this breed is not known to have a "guard dog" mentality.

HOUNDS

Hound breeds were bred to hunt and are divided into two groups, the scent followers and the sight hunters. Notable scent followers include beagles and bloodhounds; sight hunters or "gaze hounds" include greyhounds and wolfhounds. Hounds generally have a placable disposition and make good family dogs that get along well in Florida's insect-fraught warm climate. Many of the hound breeds have droopy, hanging ears, which in Florida can harbor insect parasites and therefore need to be kept clean and dry.

Afghan hounds are immediately identifiable by their tall, slender, graceful forms and elegantly silken long coats. At the shoulder, an Afghan hound stands 25 inches or more. The breed is slim, like the greyhound, weighing usually between 50 and 60 pounds. The Afghan's Egyptian origins are disputed in many dog references, but nearly all agree that the breed was perfected and named for its Afghanistan homeland. Because their coats demand considerable upkeep, these dogs often are kept only as status symbols. Few rarely get an opportunity to perform their instinctive hunting chores.

American foxhounds surfaced about three hundred years ago from English foxhound stock, which is believed to have developed from French hounds that were used in packs to hunt fox and other game in the 1300s. These foxhounds have a characteristic short coat that is black, white, and tan, and they stand about 21 to 24 inches at the shoulder. Weight is generally 55 to 65 pounds.

Basenjis are the barkless wonders of the canine world. They do not offer a typical dog yap but instead emit something like a whine or yodel. They are chipper dogs, about 17 inches at the shoulder and weighing about 23 pounds. This breed's coat is short, in variations of reddish-brown, black, or black and tan marked with white. They are sometimes not recognized as hounds because rather than having

Scientific advances in the production of frozen canine semen have been ongoing since 1969 when the first puppies conceived by frozen semen were born. Freezing techniques have improved and semen is remaining much more potent. The notion that a long-dead champion dog could continue to produce litters of highbred pups excites many breeders. But the technique is far from foolproof because female dogs are often difficult to inseminate artificially with any high degree of success.

typically long ears, a basenji's ears are upright and alert. This breed is renowned for its energy and its unflagging affection for children.

Basset hounds, with their sad eyes and long body frame atop short legs, are among the most recognizable of dogs. Actually, a basset's stubby frame is one of the most solid in the dog world, which makes this hound ideal for hunting in heavy cover. The basset generally stands just 12 to 15 inches at the shoulder while weighing 25 to 50 pounds. These dogs have a tendency to gain weight so their diets should be monitored carefully. Their compact size and excellent dispositions, however, make them good family pets in suburban settings. They fare well in Florida, too, because their coat, usually a variation of black, tan, and white, is short.

Beagles are renowned as dependable family pets, and they often rank among the most popular dogs in owner opinion surveys. They were first developed as rabbit-hunting dogs in England. Beagles have shorthaired coats generally of three colors—black, white, and brown (or tan). The breed has a compact build, in two sizes: the 13-inch version and the 15-inch model. Weight is generally from 20 to 40 pounds, although some individuals can grow obese quite easily. Beagles make excellent canine Floridians.

Bloodhounds are not often seen in cities because they can grow rather large for the average urban or suburban back yard. These dogs "sing bass," having a deep voice that carries for miles. They often are used as police tracking dogs because they have great noses, both in size and acuity. One such dog is said to have caught a prisoner after the escapee's trail was 105 hours old. Bloodhounds generally stand about 25 inches at the shoulder and weigh between 80 and 110 pounds. Their coat, while shorthaired and smooth, appears to be too large for the dog it is intended to fit. As a result, the folds of skin, as well as the ears, can harbor parasites and must be kept clean and dry. This breed's coloring ranges from combinations of black and tan, or red and tan, to solid beigy-tan.

Dachshunds are noble, perky little canines that in no way deserve to be dubbed "wiener dogs." Rarely exceeding 5 to 9 inches at the shoulder and weighing only 5 to 20 pounds, this breed makes an ideal indoor pet. Varieties of dachshunds include smooth-coated, wirehaired, and longhaired—plus miniature versions of each. Colors are black or chocolate accented with tan markings, or a solid liver-red. Coat length is not critical with this breed because most Florida dachshunds are kept indoors where temperature, insects, and humidity can be regulated. The breed, however, is somewhat prone to skin problems. Dachshunds originated in Germany centuries ago. In German, *dachs* translates to "badger" and *hund* to "dog." Thus, these "badger dogs" can be scrappy, but they are more frequently described by their owners as loving pets that make excellent watchdogs for the yard, condominium, or apartment.

Greyhounds have long been sleek status symbols among dog enthusiasts. An ancient breed dating back some 5,000 years, greyhounds were used for sport and hunt in Egypt and became a sensation in England as early as the ninth century. During Henry VII's reign, the greyhound became his badge and continues today in England as the symbol of the king's messengers. Greyhounds are tall, standing about 26 inches at the shoulder. Their aerodynamic frame is slim, with a typical greyhound weight being just 60 to 70 pounds. This breed comes in virtually every color, and the coat is short and smooth. Today, greyhounds are used extensively for racing, with many Florida cities having pari-mutuel tracks where bettors may wager on the dogs. Numerous greyhound lovers have made good pets of retired racing dogs, but some expert greyhound handlers do not agree that just anyone should enter such a venture. The experts point out racing dogs generally are not treated as pets during their early years and therefore can have difficulty adjusting to domestic life. Greyhounds should never be kept as apartment dogs for they demand exercise and plenty of space to periodically rev up to speed.

Whippets resemble small greyhounds and are said to have been an early cross between the Italian greyhound and a terrier. They are growing in popularity, although they have been favorites in England since the mid-1700s for hunting rabbits. Height of whippets is from 18 to 22 inches at the shoulder, and weight is 10 to 20 pounds. Whippets are usually white, gray, or tan. They continue to be used for racing in some regions but do make fine Florida pets because of their compact size. If kept indoors, however, they should be regularly exercised.

TERRIERS

The dog world of terriers literally began from the ground up. The term *terrier* means "earth dog" and derives from the Latin *terra*. The breed was crossed and perfected to hunt down and wrest from their hiding places small rodents and game. Even today, while few of Florida's terrier breeds ever see an actual rat or rabbit, they instinctively chase down moving toys and "kill" them with a hefty shake. Terriers generally are small dogs, although the Airedale and the Kerry blue breeds are exceptions. Terriers are easy to care for and shed less than other breeds because of their naturally close-cropped or wiry coats. Few breeds are as scrappy as terriers and they often behave a bit cocky on their leash—seeming to think they can whip any Rottweiler on the block. They make superbly devoted pets and pay for their keep with affection and by warning off any would-be intruders with displays of aggression that belie their sometimes pint size.

Airedale terriers are largest of the terriers. They stand about 23 inches at the shoulder and weigh between 40 and 50 pounds. Their tightly wiry coat is tan and black. These dogs were originally bred in a region of England around the Aire River and have long been popular with British dog owners. Airedales staunchly stand their ground and are fiercely devoted to their owners. In Florida, the Airedale fares well as long as it has sufficient exercise space.

Bedlington terriers resemble lambs but are said to possess the bravery of a lion. Their inner coat is fleecy-looking curl that is popular in the show ring and most evident after they have had their outer coats trimmed. Coat colors include white, creamy-brown, blue, and liver-red, and may be accented with tan markings. Height of this breed is 15 to 17 inches at the shoulder and weight is 17 to 23 pounds. These savvy little canines make good Florida pets and provide an able "first alert" should prowlers lurk.

Bull terriers originated in England when bulldogs and terrier breeds were crossed. The result was a breed that stands about 22 inches at the shoulder and weighs from 30 to 36 pounds. The breed was used for dogfighting in England in the 1800s, and some references cite this as the "gladiator breed." One bull terrier gained fame as the companion of U.S. General George Patton, and television advertising featuring one bull terrier "party dog" has prompted an upswing in its popularity.

Cairn terriers originated on the Isle of Skye off western Scotland. As hunting dogs, these terriers got their name for hunting among "cairn," which are rock piles used as landmarks. The breed is small, measuring just 10 inches at the shoulder and weighing 14 pounds. It sports a durable, double coat of somewhat harsh outer fur and a soft undercoat in virtually every color but white. Cairn terriers reside nicely in Florida apartments.

Fox terriers are long-legged and come in two models: wirehaired and flat-coated. Both are generally white with tan and black markings. These dogs are lively and alert as befits an animal bred in the 1800s to dig wily foxes from their dens. The size of a fox terrier is usually about 15 inches at the shoulder, and it grows to weigh between 15 and 19 pounds. Obesity is rarely a problem with these terriers because they are bundles of energy.

Miniature schnauzers are classed as terriers, unlike their giant and standard-sized cousins that belong to the working dog class. Miniatures of the breed are compact little live wires, standing just 12 to 14 inches at the shoulder and weighing 13 to 15 pounds. Coloring of these dogs, like the larger schnauzers, is black, silvery-gray, or a "salt-and-pepper" combination. Miniature schnauzers survive well in Florida, and owners report that these dogs are enjoyable apartment roommates.

Scottish terriers, or "Scotties," originated during the mid-1800s in Scotland and were used to hunt small game, including badgers. This breed is small in stature but large in nerve and verve. They stand only about 10 inches at the shoulder and weigh from 19 to 22 pounds.

They have a wiry coat that can be groomed to smoothness, and their endearing eyebrows and mustache give them a wizened expression. Whether on a Florida farm or in a Florida apartment, the Scottie is intelligent, expressive, and devoted.

Skye terriers are another of the Scottish terriers developed to ferret out small game in a climate that can be considerably harsher than Florida's. The Isle of Skye, original home of these dogs, lies off the western coast of Scotland. Skye terriers stand about 10 inches at the shoulder and feature a double coat in almost every color.

PIT BULLDOGS

The pit bulldog breed deserves special attention as an increasing number of municipalities pass laws to restrict the numbers and activities of these dogs. In Florida's Dade County, pit bulldog owners must register their dogs, keep the animals confined, post a "dangerous dog" sign, and must carry liability insurance in case their dogs attack someone. Not surprisingly, owners of pit bulldogs resent the singling out of their dog breed and are fighting the ordinance.

Besides the "discrimination" cited by pit bulldog owners is another argument: just what, precisely, is a pit bulldog? Generally, it is a dog type that resembles the American pit bull terrier or the Staffordshire terrier. The hallmark of those breeds is a sturdy physique with a particularly powerful head, neck, and chest. The American pit bull terrier is an AKC-recognized breed, as is the Staffordshire terrier. Both breeds trace back to English bulldogs and Manchester terriers.

An unregistered, more generic type of pit bulldog can be found in or behind urban homes or as regular passengers in the pickup trucks of rural Floridians. At first glance, these dogs resemble the American pit bull terrier, but many are mutts—indiscriminate crosses between pit bulldog-type animals and other dog breeds such as Rottweilers or even Great Danes.

The Staffordshire terrier breed has long been prized in England for its bravery. This breed traditionally was bred to assist farmers and hunters. With their strong jaws and powerful necks and chests, these dogs could keep hold of a farmer's errant bull or a hunter's wild boar dinner.

Prior to the 1850s, when dogfighting was legal in many of the states of this country, Staffordshire terriers, or their crosses, gained favor in dogfighting pits and the generalized "pit bulldog" was developed. Today, of course, dogfights are illegal in Florida. But this cruel blood "sport" persists in some rural areas of the state. Owning a champion fighting dog spells illicit profits and promotes the crossbreeding and inbreeding of ferocious dogs. The most valued fighting pit bulldog is strong, durable, aggressive, and, above all, refuses to release its biting hold on an opponent. Dogs in the pit fight to the death, or nearly so. Losing dogs, if not killed during the fight, often are destroyed by their owners after the fight, either because the dog is badly mangled or because the owner is disgusted with the animal.

Puppies of these fighting dogs may not display particularly ferocious tendencies. Rather, aggressive personalities are enhanced through training. The dogs are "baited" with other dogs or with dead animals. The pups are given rubber hoses to chew to strengthen jaw muscles. Stamina and muscle are built by long hours of running on treadmills.

Owners of bona fide American pit bull terriers protest the bad name their breed has received. They say their breed is a loyal, friendly animal with a gentle disposition that has been smeared by the media, which fails to report attacks by other dog breeds.

However, statistics kept by law enforcement agencies, dog-control personnel, humane associations, and the federal Center for Disease Control in Atlanta do not stack up in favor of loosening control over pit bulldogs. In 1986, for instance, the Humane Society of the United States found that pit bulldogs or their crosses accounted for 58 percent of all the dog-attack fatalities. The Center for Disease Control reported in 1989 that approximately 157 fatalities occurred from dog bites in the past decade, and that pit bulldogs accounted for more than 40 percent of those deaths. At the same time, pit bulldog-type animals accounted for less than 1 percent of the total dog population.

Humane society and dog shelter spokespersons maintain that the stigma will persist until breeders begin policing themselves. "Too many pit bulldog owners take pride in their dog's ferocious reputation," said one humane society director. "They see a pit bulldog not as a pet but as an automatic weapon." Indeed, news sources report that more drug dealers around the nation are using pit bulldogs as personal bodyguards and to guard drug stashes.

Breeders of the AKC-recognized American pit bull terriers can ultimately restore their breed's reputation. As one humane society official said, "German shepherds and Doberman pinschers had bad reputations for a while, when they were being bred as guard dogs. That changed when breeders began breeding for good temperament."

TOY BREEDS

These diminutive breeds are ideal for any home setting in Florida. Many toy breeds, such as the Pekingese, have always been small animals. Others, such as the toy poodle, originated through selective breeding of small standard-sized poodles. Most dog experts agree that it is the toy dog classification that most accurately meets the definition of "pet" because these littlest canines are smart, affectionate, and easily kept or transported. Sometimes denigrated as "yappy" by enthusiasts of larger dog breeds, these half-pints provide a perfect "alarm system" for their owners. Toys most often are owned by adults and may not have much exposure to children; as a result, perhaps because of their small size, adult-owned toy dogs are occasionally snappy with youngsters. These breeds generally are most endearing if they are exposed to playful tots while still puppies.

Chihuahuas are immediately recognizable by their oversized ears and eyes and their small body size. Weighing anywhere from 1 to 6 pounds, these small pets stand only about 5 inches at the shoulder. Hardy, affectionate, and intelligent, Chihuahuas are believed to have originated in China and from there traveled to Mexico with Spaniards sometime after the fall of the Aztec civilization. Besides the hairless variety, there are shorthaired and longhaired versions of this breed.

Maltese, with their fine coat of silken white hair and black button noses and eyes, are favorites among Florida's apartment dwellers. In fact, the Maltese's ancestors may have enjoyed similar popularity among Greek and Roman city dwellers. Standing just 5 inches at the shoulder and weighing 4 to 6 pounds, these little dogs are the essence of pampered house pets.

Papillons are occasionally confused with longhaired Chihuahuas because of their similar appearance. The papillons, called "dwarf spaniels" in the sixteenth century, are usually slightly larger than Chihuahuas, and measure between 8 and 11 inches at the shoulder.

They weigh 3 to 6 pounds. These dogs are members of the spaniel family and generally sport black and white coats, occasionally with a touch of tan. Hardy and companionable, papillons do well as indoor dogs in the state.

Pekingese date back to the eighth century where they were favorites of Chinese emperors. The breed's name translates to "lion dog." The breed became popular in Britain during the mid-1800s. "Pekes" have long, luxuriant coats that require some upkeep to stay flowing and silky. The breed, which weighs under 14 pounds, is characterized by large eyes and a turned-up pug nose. Fiercely devoted to the family, Pekes make good watchdogs for yard and apartment. They should not be kept outdoors in Florida's heat.

Pomeranians are another of the fluffy toy breeds. Resembling miniature foxes, this breed has large, expressive eyes, a pointed snout, and perky little upright ears. A pomeranian's double coat favors cool climes, probably because the breed descended from breeds found in Iceland and Lapland. Fortunately, a pomeranian's small size means it can enjoy air-conditioned indoor life and rarely suffer in Florida. Specimens rarely weigh more than 7 pounds and are seen in virtually any solid coat color. Their popularity soared during Queen Victoria's reign because she favored the breed.

Pugs have often been depicted in paintings of aristocracy and are thought to date back to 400 B.C. The breed is compact, sturdy, close-coated, and characterized by prominent dark eyes with a turned-up pug nose. Coloring is most often silver or apricot, and weight rarely exceeds 18 pounds. Intelligent and affectionate, pugs are ideal Florida house pets, although their wrinkly skin may occasionally need special attention.

Shih tzus enjoy a noble ancestry. Prized by the Chinese emperors in the 1500s, it is believed they were a gift from the Tibetan Dali Lamas to the Chinese emperors. This breed sports a longhaired coat of any color, which requires daily grooming. But it is worth the trouble because these attractive and affectionate dogs fit so nicely in any household. Slightly larger than some toy breeds, shih tzus measure 8 to 11 inches at the shoulder and weigh 12 to 15 pounds. The name translates from Chinese as "lion son dog."

Toy poodles are the tiniest of the three poodle sizes. They weigh about 6 pounds and stand no more than 10 inches at the shoulder. Fashionably clipped or not, these dogs have a coat that sheds little and requires almost no upkeep. Toy poodles are lively and smart, making a chic addition to any Florida dwelling. (See also Poodles in the "Nonsporting Breeds" section.)

Yorkshire terriers rank among the smallest terriers, but they are typical terriers—spirited and scrappy. "Yorkies" are but 9 inches at the shoulder and weigh up to 7 pounds. Their glorious blue-gray coat is long and fine and generally accented with tan markings. Such small dogs obviously belong indoors, and Yorkies make superb apartment dogs. Their silky coat demands some grooming time, but most Yorkie owners find it a delightful chore. These dogs originated in the Yorkshire region of England in the mid-1800s.

NONSPORTING BREEDS

This dog classification, sometimes called companion dogs, is widely varied. Most members of this group were previously working or hunting dogs but today are primarily considered pets.

Boston terriers originated in the United States when bulldogs and white terriers were crossed during the mid-1800s. These dogs make ideal city dogs. They have short, close coats of brindle or black with white markings. Weight is usually between 13 and 25 pounds, with a height of between 14 and 17 inches at the shoulder. Boston terriers are active little dogs that display much affection yet fearlessly guard the homestead.

Bulldogs, with their characteristically flattened nose, always appear grumpy. Indeed, the breed has a history of use in Britain for bullbaiting or pit fighting. The bulldog's short, fine-textured coat is white, fawn, brindle, and occasionally red. As a successful fighting breed, it is built with a low center of gravity. The usual bulldog stands just 15 inches at the shoulder, yet weighs a hefty 40 to 50 pounds.

Chow Chows sometimes have a difficult time finding much comfort in Florida's heat unless they are clipped or kept indoors in air conditioning. This breed originated in China some 2,000 years ago, where it was used for hunting. A dense, double coat of fur tends to stand out from the animal's body, lending it a bearlike appearance.

This is a powerful breed, which stands 19 to 23 inches at the shoulder and weighs 50 to 60 pounds. Owners and veterinarians report that this breed tends to be very protective of its home territory and is best kept confined unless it is well disciplined.

Dalmatians are easily among the most recognizable of dog breeds with their white coats sprinkled with either brown or black dots. The origin of the breed is murky, although it is thought to have developed in Dalmatia, a part of Yugoslavia. These dogs traditionally served as coach dogs and continue today as mascots of some fire departments. Dalmatians grow to a height of 19 to 23 inches at the shoulder and weigh between 35 and 50 pounds. They are excellent companion dogs and make dependable watchdogs.

Lhasa apsos are gaining popularity in Florida because they make ideal indoor pets. They are small, just 10 inches at the shoulder, and weigh only 13 to 15 pounds. Lhasas have a long, silky coat of any imaginable color that requires some regular grooming. The breed developed in Tibet centuries ago.

Poodles also are popular in this state—their beauty, brains, and easy upkeep make them ideal Floridians. Poodles come in three sizes: standard, miniature, and toy. The standard poodle is the largest, weighing up to 55 pounds with a shoulder height of over 15 inches. Miniature versions stand 15 inches (with a 10-inch minimum) at the shoulder and weigh about 15 pounds. Toys stand 10 inches or less. The breed originally was used as a retriever, and the different types of "high-fashioned" clips reflect this outdoor heritage; hair was shaved off, or left on, to provide optimum protection for the dog in the field. Derivation of the breed's name is the German *pudel*, short for *pudelhund* (or "puddle-dog").

HERDING BREEDS

Herding dogs have a time-honored heritage of helping their owners move livestock from one location to another. Like the working breed group, herding dogs often display a businesslike attitude, and are nearly impossible to distract while they are tending sheep or cattle. Even citified individuals in this group may continue exhibiting herding instincts with ducks at a neighborhood pond, other family pets, or even passing vehicles. Indeed, while any dog breed can acquire the dangerous habit of chasing cars, herding dogs seem especially prone to trying to round up passing autos, bicyclists, and motorcycles. Beauty, brains, and faithfulness are hallmarks of this dog group.

The **collie** is among the best known of the herding breed group. It is immediately recognized as the "Lassie" dog. And, as that famous dog's name suggests, the breed is of Scottish origins, bred to herd sheep. The collie can stand 22 to 26 inches at the shoulder and weigh 50 to 75 pounds. Collies come in two coat types: rough-coated (like Lassie), and smooth-coated. They come in a variety of colors, ranging from white or blue merle, to sable and white, to a blend of mostly black with white markings and tan shadings.

German shepherds are renowned for their quick intelligence. This breed is sturdy, standing about 25 inches at the shoulder and carrying between 60 and 85 pounds. A shepherd's coat is usually black, gray, or tan and black, and a few individuals are white. Because it has a diligent, obedient nature, the German shepherd strives to please. It can be counted on to do whatever it is asked, and has become a popular addition to police work and in guiding sightless humans.

Old English sheepdogs are, as the name implies, sheep-herding animals developed primarily in England during the 1800s. They are lovably bulky dogs with a shoulder height of 22 inches and up and a weight of 55 to 65 pounds. Because this breed often is exuberant, affectionate, and cuddly-looking, it is difficult to remember that it is also a dedicated herding dog and happiest when given some task, if only catching a Frisbie. The coat of the sheepdog is a shaggy, dense, double layer of fur; it is generally gray, blue, or blue-merle, and may or may not be accented with white markings. Some veterinarians do not recommend Florida as home to this breed because of its dense fur covering. Many sheepdogs suffer from Florida's humidity and insects, prompting owners to give them a comfortable clip.

Shetland sheepdogs, also called "Shelties," resemble what could be termed miniature collies. They originated in the Shetland Islands north of Scotland. Shelties are rather small dogs, just 13 to 16 inches at the shoulder, and weigh about 15 pounds. Developed by shepherds in the nineteenth century, this breed is designed for the cold outdoors with its double coat of silken black, blue-merle, or sable, with tan and/or white accents. Shelties are intelligent and quick to learn, but as with other herding breeds, they can soon learn to replace their love of corraling sheep with chasing vehicles. This breed is small enough for apartments or urban back yards, and can be comfortable in Florida if kept in air conditioning or clipped during the summertime.

Welsh Corgis are among the smallest of herding dogs and, by accounts dating back to 1200 B.C., among the oldest of British Isle breeds. Extremely pleasant natured, this breed is built low and long— only 10 to 12 inches tall, yet 36 to 44 inches long, and weighing about 26 pounds. There are two types of Corgis, the tailless Pembroke and the short-tailed Cardigan. They were used in Britain to nip at the heels of livestock, not for herding their owner's livestock so much as for herding away the neighbor's intruding livestock. Colors of Corgis include red, sable, fawn, black-and-tan, all with or without white markings.

OTHER BREED SELECTION CONSIDERATIONS

It cannot be overemphasized that heavily furred dog breeds may not remain in top health in Florida. Many owners report that by air conditioning the dog's habitat (inside or outside) and by virtually shearing the coat, these breeds can be kept comfortable. Such steps, however, can add to the cost and time of keeping such dogs.

Similarly, all large dog breeds must have adequate living space and are not appropriate selections for the average mobile home park, apartment, or condominium.

Persons considering the purchase of dogs that will mature at more than 25 pounds should also be aware that some breeds are prone to develop hip dysplasia, also called subluxation in some texts. The ailment develops gradually in dogs that may appear perfectly normal. Many owners first discover this ailment when their Great Dane, German shepherd, Rottweiler, or other sturdy dog breed begins displaying stiffness or pain when it moves quickly or jumps up. Thought to be hereditary, the disease occurs when the ball-like femoral head of the hind leg stops fitting properly into the hip socket.

Calcium deposits form and the area grows increasingly deformed. Eventually, the capsule that holds the two bones together may rupture and the pet must be humanely destroyed.

The only effective way of dealing with hip dysplasia at this time is to not breed dogs that are prone to the disease. Any large breed of dog being considered for breeding should be X-rayed by a veterinarian.

In addition to hip dysplasia, German shepherds are apt to get another ailment, degenerative myelopathy, a nerve disease that behaves like human multiple sclerosis. The fatal disease is estimated to affect more than half of all German shepherds between the ages of six and fourteen years. Research is underway at the University of Florida's College of Veterinary Medicine to find a cure through drugs. Meanwhile, reports from the Veterinary College indicate success with the use of aminocaproic acid (EACA). This medication has been used since 1980 and has effectively slowed the deterioration of affected dogs. EACA is costly, however, and must be given to the dog for the rest of its life.

Washington, D.C., is the largest user of police dogs. The Capitol Police Department, the Secret Service, the Metropolitan Police Department, the U.S. Park Police, and the Smithsonian Institution all keep a coterie of canines walking the beat.

Favored for police work are male German shepherds from one to three years of age. Cost of training the dogs runs $5,000 to $8,000 and takes fourteen weeks. Training includes obedience, agility, tracking, and searching buildings.

In addition, roving Rovers routinely watch over some of Washington, D.C.'s most revered sites, including the thirteen popular museums operated by the Smithsonian Institution. The museum complex, which contains an estimated 134 million items, is patrolled by its own canine corps that ferrets out everything from lost wallets to the occasional pickpocket. The dogs also sniff out persons who linger behind after museum doors have closed.

The following reference chart is designed to assist prospective dog purchasers in making a selection. This is not a complete list, but it does include many of the most popular breeds.

Chart Codes:

Size: (S) Breeds of under 20 pounds
          (M) Breeds of from 20 to 45 pounds
          (L) Breeds of 45 pounds and up

Recommended Living Space:
          (A) Ideal apartment-sized dogs
          (O) Adapts to outdoor yards
          (E) Extra exercise room recommended

Coat Type: (S) Shorthaired, smooth or curly
            (M) Moderate length that may require some grooming
                 or clipping
            (L) Densely longhaired

SPORTING BREEDS

Breed	Size	Space	Coat
Golden Retriever	(L)	(O)(E)	(M)
Labrador Retriever	(L)	(O)(E)	(S)
Chesapeake Bay Retriever	(L)	(O)(E)	(S)
Brittany Spaniel	(L)	(O)(E)	(M)
Cocker Spaniel	(M)	(A)	(M)
English Springer Spaniel	(L)	(O)(E)	(M)
English Setter	(L)	(O)(E)	(M)
Gordon Setter	(L)	(O)(E)	(M)
Irish Setter	(L)	(O)(E)	(M)
German Wirehaired Pointer	(L)	(O)(E)	(S)
German Shorthaired Pointer	(L)	(O)(E)	(S)
Wirehaired Pointing Griffon	(L)	(O)(E)	(S)
Weimaraner	(L)	(O)(E)	(S)

WORKING BREEDS

Breed	Size	Space	Coat
Alaskan Malamute	(L)	(O)(E)	(L)
Boxer	(L)	(O)(E)	(D)
Doberman Pinscher	(L)	(O)(E)	(S)
Great Dane	(L)	(E)	(S)
Rottweiler	(L)	(O)(E)	(S)
St. Bernard	(L)	(O)(E)	(L)
Samoyed	(L)	(O)(E)	(M)
Schnauzer, Giant	(L)	(O)(E)	(M)
Schnauzer, Standard	(M)	(O)(E)	(M)
Siberian Husky	(M-L)	(O)(E)	(L)

HOUND BREEDS

Breed	Size	Space	Coat
Afghan	(L)	(O)(E)	(L)
American Foxhound	(L)	(O)(E)	(S)
Basenji	(M)	(A)(O)	(S)
Basset	(M-L)	(A)(O)	(S)
Beagle	(M)	(A)(O)	(S)
Bloodhound	(L)	(O)(E)	(S)
Dachshund	(S)	(A)	(S)(M)
Greyhound	(L)	(O)(E)	(S)
Whippet	(L)	(A)(O)	(S)

TERRIERS

Breed	Size	Space	Coat
Airedale	(M-L)	(O)(E)	(M)
Bedlington	(M)	(A)(O)	(M)
Bull	(M)	(A)(O)	(S)
Cairn	(S)	(A)(O)	(M)
Fox	(S)	(A)(O)	(S)(M)
Scottish	(S-M)	(A)(O)	(M)
Skye	(S)	(A)	(L)

NONSPORTING BREEDS

Breed	Size	Space	Coat
Boston Terrier	(S)	(A)(O)	(S)
Bulldog	(L)	(O)	(S)
Chow Chow	(L)	(O)(E)	(L)
Dalmatian	(M-L)	(O)(E)	(S)
Lhasa Apso	(S)	(A)	(M)
Poodle, Standard	(L)	(O)(E)	(M)
Poodle, Miniature	(S)	(A)	(M)

HERDING BREEDS

Breed	Size	Space	Coat
Collie	(L)	O)(E)	(S)(M)
German Shepherd	(L)	(O)(E)	(M)
Old English Sheepdog	(L)	(O)(E)	(L)
Shetland Sheepdog	(S)	(A)(O)	(M)
Welsh Corgi	(M)	(A)(O)	(M)

TOY

Breed	Size	Space	Coat
Chihuahua	(S)	(A)	(S)(M)
Maltese	(S)	(A)	(L)
Papillon	(S)	(A)	(S)
Pekingese	(S)	(A)	(M)
Pomeranian	(S)	(A)	(M)
Poodle	(S)	(A)	(M)
Pug	(S)	(A)	(S)
Shih Tzu	(S)	(A)	(L)
Yorkshire Terrier	(S)	(A)	(L)

When a man's dog turns against him it is time for his wife to pack her trunk and go home to mamma.
                    —Mark Twain

CHAPTER 3

Make Room for Doggie

THE OUTDOOR LIFE

Appropriate housing for a dog in Florida is a must. Granted, winters are mild except in the most northern regions of the state where frost, even occasional snow, occurs from Gainesville north into the Panhandle. It is from the long, blistering days of summer that Florida dogs must be protected.

The warmest months are July, August, and September, when daytime temperatures average anywhere from 80 degrees in the northern portions of the state to 84 degrees in the Keys. Again, those are averages. A dog tied outside in direct summer sun will spend several hours exposed to temperatures closer to 115 degrees. Such cruel neglect is sufficient grounds for authorities to impound the dog, especially if the animal is found to be without water.

In addition, Florida is the thunderstorm capital of the United States, consistently leading the nation in human deaths due to lightning. And within the state, the Tampa Bay area tallies the most days of thunderstorm activity, about 120 per year. As a result, many dogs in Florida develop a fear of the booming storms that borders on blind panic. The outdoor dog should never be chained to the only tall tree in the yard; that is tantamount to tying Spot to a lightning rod. A study of lightning-caused injuries and deaths to humans from 1959 to 1985 revealed that 29 percent of those incidents occurred near trees.

Thus, it is simply a humane consideration for owners to provide their dogs with a safe haven from Florida's heat and rain. And if climate and weather are not reason enough, providing shelter for a dog kept outdoors is also state law.

A shelter does not have to be a fancy air-conditioned or carpeted castle. A roofed structure or enclosed porch is sufficient. The shelter should be clean and roomy enough to accommodate the dog when it is lying down and have enough head room for the dog to stand up.

Ideally, a doghouse should be built with the following considerations in mind:

—It should be up off the ground a few inches. Many Florida days and nights are humid, so providing space between the ground and the dog's resting place promotes air circulation.

—A watertight roof will keep the doghouse interior dry and warmer in winter months. Keeping the interior dry also discourages mildewing and helps ward off skin diseases.

—A ledge on which food and water dishes can be set will prevent the dog from knocking them over and making a mess. Most dogs will not sleep in a dirty house, so bug-infested filth is, from Rover's standpoint, an eviction notice.

—By nature, a dog is curious and generally craves human attention; therefore, a dog is most comfortable when his house and enclosure are constructed so that he can watch what is going on in or around the house. If the dog is expected to bark at intruders, then it is necessary to place him where he can see and be heard.

Once the doghouse is built, it can be placed inside a fenced enclosure large enough to permit the dog to get exercise. A good rule of thumb is to make the enclosure two times the dog's body length in width and four to six times the dog's body length (include the tail) in lengthwise roominess. This means that for a medium-large dog, one forty-five inches from nose to tail, a good-sized enclosure would measure eight feet by twenty feet.

Some dog owners and breeders prefer to make at least part of the

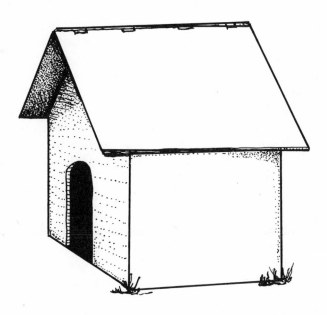

The traditional doghouse. Although not visible, the floor is built up from the ground. The roof is hinged to open for cleaning.

run out of concrete because it is easy to wash down and helps to keep Fido clean. At least a portion of any concrete run should be shaded. Otherwise, it will be too hot for the dog to use during summer.

Materials other than concrete may be used, but while less expensive to install, they do have their drawbacks. One option is to leave the area covered by grass, but keep in mind that runs built on grass may quickly turn to sand in Florida's heat. Then, with one downpour, the quarters become muddy wallows. Other materials such as clay or limestone provide good drainage, but these runs can become colorfully dusty, may be dug up or under by the dog, and will need periodic replacing.

There are advantages to being able to keep the dog outdoors. For one, the owner's home is less likely to be infested with fleas (although the insects can be carried in by humans from the dog's area). Also, the necessity of paper training the dog is eliminated.

Disadvantages also exist. Foremost is that an "out-of-sight" phenomenon often occurs, and the dog interacts less with the family. As a result, some lonesome dogs initiate bad habits to get attention. Barking and digging are the most common misbehaviors that prompt many disgruntled owners to get rid of their dogs.

Another frequent complaint heard by persons who keep their dogs penned most of the time is that the dog does not behave itself when freed from the pen. Cooped-up canines tend to run off, jump up on people, and generally act out of control. Such behavior is not the dog's fault. It's simply a natural canine reaction to unaccustomed freedom. A dog needs to be unpenned each day, handled, groomed, walked, played with—and loved.

A second drawback to keeping a dog outdoors, particularly in Florida, is that the animal is apt to be more bothered by insects such as mites and fleas, more susceptible to skin diseases such as fungus, and more exposed to mosquitoes that in Florida transmit the all-too-common heartworm. Regular cleaning of the dog's house and run is crucial, as is keeping up the outdoor dog's heartworm preventative.

THE INDOOR DOG

Oh, for the life of a pampered Palm Beach poodle whose polished nails rarely touch anything rougher than carpeting. Viewing such a coddled animal makes one forget that it is a dog, not a person. Living in such an artificial climate is not a lifestyle nature intended for a dog; dry heat in winter as well as dry cooling all summer can take a toll on the pampered dog's coat.

Another downside to housing the pooch inside is that the living quarters must be vacuum cleaned more often to keep shedded dog hairs from forming dust bunnies the size of Cleveland. There is also the disadvantage of the dog having to be paper trained and walked outside on a leash for nature calls.

Boredom also affects indoor dogs, especially those whose owners work all day and enjoy arriving home late. If left alone for long hours, a housebound pup is more likely to have accidents. Boredom also builds bad habits. An example is the case of one dog who literally ate all the vinyl flooring from the tiny bathroom where he was kept all day while his mistress was away earning the dog food. Another confined lonely dog wailed and howled until the neighbors' complaints forced the owner to give the dog away.

Keeping the dog (especially a small breed) inside does have its merits. Fido stays cleaner, more free of fleas. And some indoor dogs have never seen a tick. Another plus is that of home protection: law enforcement officials say burglaries are less apt to occur in homes or apartments that contain barking dogs.

Dogs kept inside may be cleaner, but owners tend to overbathe their canine roommates. Skin problems caused by dry skin or blow-drying occur, and thus the cleanest dog may scratch just as it would if it had a flea infestation. Surprisingly, the ever-inside dog also may develop flea dermatitis because the dog encounters insect pests so infrequently that it develops no natural immunity to flea bites.

If kept indoors, the dog should have a place of its own. A washable foam doghouse or a simple cushion gives the dog a secure place to go if its owners are not home, a thunderstorm rolls in, or if the children, grandchildren, or a brassy cat gets too cheeky.

If the household is climate controlled, place the dog's bed out of drafts. Corners provide cozy niches that are rarely in the line of an air vent. Some dogs prefer their bed to be near where the owner sleeps; others enjoy being in the middle of things and are most happy to sneak into the owner's bed whenever the getting is good.

Some dogs have the best of both worlds, living both indoors and out. They may sleep indoors at night and come in and out of the house during the day. Such arrangements only work if the owner is at home all day or if the owner installs a doggie door. While this system makes for very contented dogs, it tends to make the indoor flea problem more acute. Owners have to vacuum the house more often and must keep Fido bathed regularly.

Whether a dog can be kept inside as a family member or must be housed outside depends on the particular owner's situation and, in part, on the effect of Florida's climate on the dog.

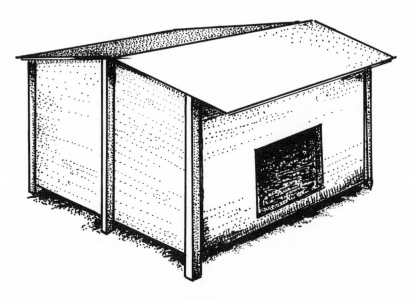

A good house for a large breed of dog. Sturdy and built up off the ground, this type of house shelters against the heat, rain, and cold. One drawback could be difficulty in cleaning this house unless the roof is built to be removed. For additional air circulation, screened vents can be placed near the roof line.

EQUIPMENT AND SUPPLIES

The dog owner, depending upon his or her pocketbook and the occasional flights of fancy, may purchase canine equipment and accessories forever. A few basics are musts, however.

Every owner's first purchase is generally some sort of restraining device—a leash—paired with either a collar or a harness. These devices are manufactured in every conceivable material from rhinestone-studded vinyl or leather, to webbed nylon or cotton, to metal chains. The well-heeled dog may even sport collars and leashes of gold plate with or without a diamond or two.

The choice of leash and collar or harness depends on several variables. The primary consideration is probably the dog's size or breed, coupled with how the device will be used. A large, strong breed needs a collar and leash to match, while a toy breed that spends much of its time indoors will likely do best wearing a lightweight collar and leash. Most dog trainers tend toward simplicity for training or exercising. A humanely-used choke chain collar in stainless steel is durable, easy to keep clean, and provides a persuasive restraint for a dog that tries muscling its owner down the sidewalk.

Every dog should become accustomed to a collar and leash as soon as possible. Soft nylon or cotton webbing provides safe, yet sturdy, starter collars for puppies. Small chain collars can also be used, but care must be taken to ensure the chain links are too tiny for the dog's teeth to fit through. Many dogs react initially to new collars by trying a Houdini-like escape trick in which they scoot the collar up and over their heads. When that happens, the dog often gets the collar about mouth-high and ends up with it in its mouth. In those circumstances, a dog can damage and even extract a tooth that gets caught in a chain link.

Once it is time to start training the dog, a choke collar is recommended by most handlers. These collars feature a ring through which the collar can be loosened or tightened depending on the pressure put on it. Because a tight collar makes the dog uncomfortable, the dog usually will yield to the collar's tightening, which then automatically loosens. Thus the dog is immediately rewarded when it does not pull on the collar. A sharp yank by the owner soon convinces the dog that if it will not pull on the collar, everyone is more comfortable.

Some owners do not like choke chains. They prefer so-called figure-eight harnesses, one end of which encircles the dog's neck while the other end encircles the dog's body behind its front legs. This works well as a restraint up to a point. If the dog is small enough, the owner can effectively keep the dog in check; if the dog is, say, a Great Dane, then the choke chain collar is probably more effective.

Trainers or breeders can recommend the best type of collar for the breed of dog that you select. All collars should have the owner's name, address, and phone number attached, in case the dog gets lost. If required by local laws, license tags should also be fastened to the collar.

Several devices are available that permit a dog to run outdoors in a confined area. Some of these attach to the ground via a long line connected to a corkscrew-type metal stake. These systems are not ideal because dogs can become tangled and injure themselves. In addition, large breeds are sometimes strong enough to pull the stake out of the ground and run off with it dragging behind and thus capable of catching on some object.

A slightly better system is a sliding ring or device that slides along an overhead cord. Even this method can present problems, however. Large dogs, if given enough slack to lie down and rest, may have enough cord in which to tangle themselves when they are standing up. Careful measuring is required to prevent this problem and still permit the dog a measured degree of freedom.

The best means of limited freedom, of course, is to build a run for the dog.

Feed and Water Bowls

Proper food and water dishes are vital items for dogs and puppies. Again, the selections available are confined only to imagination.

Stainless steel dishes maintain themselves well. They do not rust, the dog cannot chew them up, and they are easy to clean.

Because larger breeds tend to scoot their bowls around the floor, manufacturers of feed bowls have come up with several options to keep them anchored. One features a wall bracket into which the food and water bowls are fitted. But these must be fitted at the proper height or the dog will be unable to clean out all the rations. If the bracket is mounted too low, the dog may be able to dislodge the bowls from the bracket.

Another inventive manufacturer has devised bowls designed to stay in place with suction cups. Many large dogs are capable of dislodging these bowls, but they work well for smaller animals. Bowls also are designed for dogs with long ears. They are conical shaped, wide at the bottom and narrow enough at the top to keep the ears from draping into the food.

Probably the most useful food and water dishes for all sized dogs are those that are made of earthenware and shaped slightly wider at the bottom and narrower at the top. These are heavy, virtually impossible to tip over, and, if placed on a rubber mat, are difficult for the dog to move during the dining hour. Some dog-supply catalogs make these hard-glazed bowls available with personalized dog names.

In Florida, many regions have hard water, so it is important to keep the water bowl clean. And food dishes should be cleaned after every meal to keep the state's abundant insect life from invading for a share of even the most minute leftovers.

For dogs that are confined outdoors, bulk food dispensers are available. They come in various sizes, and some hold as much as fifty pounds of feed. The dog eats from a tray and additional rations slide down the dispenser to replace what has been eaten. These dispensers are available in galvanized metal and in plastic; some are equipped with automatic timers. A handy way to feed, dispensers provide some protection from moisture and insects, but there are a couple of drawbacks. One is that a greedy dog can eat until it drops. Another strike against these dispensers is that they will attract bugs that enter through the open tray.

Similarly, automatic waterers are available for dogs, whether they stay indoors or outside. These work well but must be kept cleaned of algae buildup and mineral deposits. Another drawback is that the waterers must be regularly checked and kept clean or the float valve can stick, resulting in a flood.

Bedding

Every dog needs a place to call its own. But whether it is a carrying crate fitted with a blanket or an elaborate, padded Taj Mahal, a few musts need consideration.

Primary in selecting a dog bed is cleanliness. Dog dander and the occasional flea demand that the dog bed be washed about once a

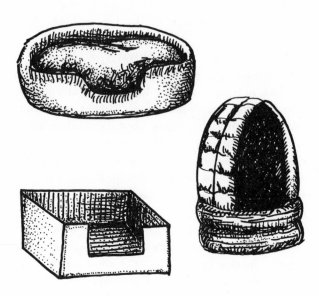

Dogs kept indoors enjoy having their own bed. Various types include the foam and pillow type, the hutch style, and for puppies, the ordinary cardboard box.

week. Fuzzy or plush materials look nice when new, but after a few launderings the fuzz gets nappy and looks dirty even when clean. Hutch-type beds are enjoyed by some dogs, especially small breeds. Even though some models feature washable covers, they can be tricky to refit on the beds after laundering.

Another dog bed features a foam semicircular shape into which a washable pillow fits. Dogs like these. But again, make sure the cover on the pillow slips off for laundering. Some models require the entire pillow be washed, and the large sizes literally take days to dry, even in a dryer.

Gaining popularity, at least with dog owners, is the cedar-chip-filled dog pillows. They consist of a bag of cedar chips and filler covered by a removable, washable outer covering. These beds are pleasingly aromatic and do seem to aid in suppressing dog odor. Some dogs do not like the red cedar odor when these beds are new—perhaps the

Breeders recommend building sand as a good surface for dog runs. It is easy to clean, keeps the dog clean, and can be easily replaced.

aroma is too strong for acute canine noses. Some manufacturers of these beds claim the cedar repels fleas, but there is no scientific evidence that such claims are valid.

Many other options exist for pet bedding, including some that claim to aid elderly or ill dogs. Although these beds bear a medical-sounding name, they are often nothing more than foam rubber available at many retail stores, covered with a fleecy pad. Still other beds offer electrical heating. Indeed, they may make outdoor dogs, or cold-natured indoor dogs, more comfortable. But these beds have plug-in electrical cords that are accessible to the dog, and any chewing on such cords could lead to electrocution or create a fire hazard.

Ironically, with the exception of some of the very largest dog breeds, the best indoor bed may be a dog crate. Made of plastic or metal wire, these devices can be closed up for carrying the dog to shows or to the veterinarian. This is handy, too, if visitors arrive and the dog becomes panicky or gets underfoot. Many dogs grow to enjoy such enclosures and view them as safe havens. Some owners toss a colorful throw over the top or a portion of the sides and the dog has its own cozy cave in which to nap or retreat from noise. Most dogs will grow to dislike crates if they are continually locked up inside of them for long hours. Owners should allow the dog to come and go freely as much as possible.

After deliberating the pros and cons of the various dog beds that are available, conclusions that most owners reach include:

1. The dog bed should be easily cleaned.
2. A bed should be roomy enough for the dog to be able to turn around and snuggle into.
3. Placement of the dog bed should be away from drafts and foot traffic.

Virtually every dog will be comfortable indoors, where the climate is controlled. Having its own bed offers a "sense of place" for the pet and contributes as much to the psychological welfare of the dog as to its physical needs.

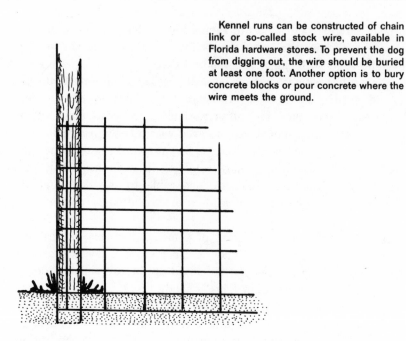

Kennel runs can be constructed of chain link or so-called stock wire, available in Florida hardware stores. To prevent the dog from digging out, the wire should be buried at least one foot. Another option is to bury concrete blocks or pour concrete where the wire meets the ground.

Toys

If there is one truth in the canine world, it is that puppies, and many adult dogs, will chew. In fact, destructive chewing is one of the prime factors leading owners to get rid of their dogs.

Puppies are compelled to chew while they are teething and exploring their new world. Because they have no hands, they tend to check out objects with their mouths. As for adult dogs, they will get in the habit of chewing if they are bored. So that is where toys come in—as alleviators of boredom for adult dogs and as aids to teething puppies.

Squeaking toys are probably not the best choice. Some dogs

tolerate noisy toys, but many dislike them, and the annoying squawks and squeaks get to many owners, too. Besides, the little noise mechanisms can fall out of the toys and be eaten or become lodged in the dog's throat. Owners often are charmed by the many appealing shapes of noisy toys—adorable little birds and mice, colorful fire hydrants and balls, all shapes that are meant to appeal to the owner, not the dog. The dog does not know it is gnawing on an itty-bitty panda bear with big blue eyes. Actually, these little toys are not a good choice for a pet. They weather, they fall apart, and the dog ends up consuming indigestible pieces of the rubber or plastic.

Far safer are the polyurethane toys, many of which are bone-shaped and flexible enough to provide good chewing yet durable enough to remain in one piece. Never purchase a toy made of any material that is small enough to fit entirely in a dog's mouth. Expert eaters that they are, canines can choke. For that matter, if the dog manages to chew a large toy down to small pieces, it is time to discard it.

Many of the best dog toys are those that both the owner and the pet can play with. Frisbies or tug-of-war pulls provide the dog (and owner) with exercise and plenty of enjoyment.

Whether your dog should be given natural bones to chew depends on the dog's habits. Some dogs aggressively attack bones and do not quit until the bone is completely eaten. Even the best of these bones can produce sharp chips and may damage the dog's teeth or gums. Always check with your veterinarian for a recommendation about which natural bones are best. Again, never give the dog a bone that is small enough to fit entirely in its mouth. It may cause choking.

Rawhide toys or chews have become very popular, but the quality of some is questionable. Cheap rawhides can contain hide material that is tainted with chemicals or even pesticides. Owners should realize that rawhide chews are not toys; dogs consider them food and will gnaw on them until they are gone. If sufficient amounts of tainted rawhide are consumed, digestive upset can be the result. So if rawhide is selected to provide chewing exercise for the dog, make sure the rawhide is top quality and is sanitized. It is a good idea to purchase such an item from a reputable pet store or from a veterinarian's office.

Accessories

Many canine-associated items can be considered accessories—nonessentials that add beauty, convenience, or effectiveness to owners' or their dogs' lives. Of course, just which items meet that definition vary. And some are more effective than others. They range from grooming appliances such as vacuum cleaners and blow dryers to dog apparel.

One of the most effective and necessary accessories is a dog nail clipper. They come in a range of sizes and costs to fit every dog and every owner's pocketbook. Clippers vary in style from pruning-shear type devices to scissors.

Coat clippers are another handy tool, although primarily needed only by persons who intend to show their dog. Before tackling a home clipping job, it is a good idea to consult a professional groomer. Although the dog's coat will grow back even after a poor clipping job, razors can occasionally cut or nick, so owners should know how to handle these items properly.

Owners who travel often with their pets might consider pet automobile safety belts that are available. They generally are made of nylon material that forms an adjustable, vestlike restraint that straps to the car's seat belt.

Similarly, life jackets are manufactured for the boating canine. Under normal circumstances, dogs are adequate swimmers, but in the event of an accident, a jacket could keep the dog from tiring before it gets plucked from the water. These must be fitted properly and should be carefully tested on the dog to make sure it aids rather than hinders the dog's ability to swim.

In the cities, where dogs are walked or kept in confined spaces, a "pooper scooper" is a handy accessory. These cleanup tools come in various sizes and materials such as plastic or metal. Some models have a scissor action; others are simply two separate pieces.

Whether for walking or simply lounging around the house, dog coats or sweaters are plentifully available for the cold-natured dog. Dogs are genetically turned out to be naturally warm in most weather, and few breeds ever shiver in Florida, so many dogs are unnecessarily "dressed" for warmth. Still, some small breeds without much of a coat, such as Chihuahuas, might be more comfortable on

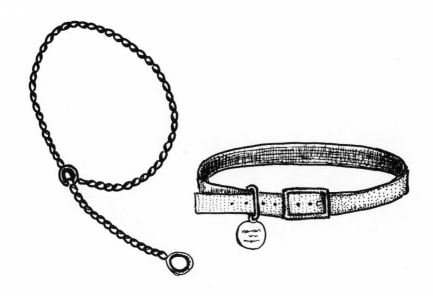

The two most popular collar styles include the choke chain (left) and the nylon web collar. A dog's rabies and identification tag should be placed on the collar if the animal goes outside.

the coldest of Florida days if they don a sweater. Other dogs that could benefit from wearing a coat or sweater on chilly days are those that are clipped for showing.

But beyond the trips outdoors on Florida's few wintry days, there is little need to keep dogs dressed. Dogs kept outdoors generally acclimate to the cooler weather and are comfortable as long as they have a house with a bed inside that affords them a windbreak and a place to curl up and retain their body heat.

Some clothing offered by dog catalogs stretches into the realm of pure anthropomorphism—attributing human characteristics to animals. The fact that dogs will permit themselves to be placed in Santa Claus suits, Halloween costumes, sloganed tee shirts, and baby clothes merely affirms the big-hearted nature of our canine friends.

> **❝**_Healing is a matter of time, but it is sometimes also a matter of opportunity._
> _—Hippocrates_ **❞**

CHAPTER 4

The Worm Turns

Warmth and moisture, two of Florida's notable climatic features, make the state a dog worm's paradise. It is under these conditions that the wriggly internal parasites thrive. Heartworms, tapeworms, hookworms, roundworms, and whipworms are the most common vitality-sapping pests that can plague Florida's canine residents. Modern veterinary medicine has made it an easy task to eradicate and prevent worms, but it takes some cooperation from an owner with know-how and diligence.

HEARTWORM

The chief life-robbing enemy of Florida dogs is heartworm. While the parasite is found in other regions of the nation, it is particularly troublesome in this state because it is borne by the mosquito, an insect that some wags suggest should be the official state animal.

The trouble begins when a mosquito bites a dog that is already infected with heartworm, which is a type of roundworm. Larvae are taken in by the mosquito, which then may pass it along to the skin of an uninfected dog. Even dogs that have been brought to Florida with their vacationing owners have been taken back home with heartworm infestation. A veterinarian in another state may not immediately recognize the problem, although the ailment is spreading rapidly.

The first step of heartworm transmission occurs when a mosquito feeds on the blood of a heartworm-infected dog. The blood contains microfilariae—microscopic-sized heartworm larvae. In about three weeks, the microfilariae develop within the mosquito into larvae capable of infecting another dog. The second step of transmission then occurs when the infected mosquito bites another dog and deposits the infective heartworm larvae on the dog's skin at the mosquito bite site. The larvae enter the dog via the opening made by the mosquito bite. Over the next two to four months, the larvae gradually migrate to the dog's heart, where they mature.

Mature heartworms can live in a dog's heart and connecting blood vessels for years. During that time, the mature female heartworm produces microfilariae that enter the dog's bloodstream, where they may be ingested by a biting mosquito and passed along to another dog. It may take years, but if left to thrive, heartworms eventually cause the animal's death.

Symptoms of heartworm infestation include gradual weight loss, an increased inability to exercise, and an exercise-induced cough. Advanced cases display increased temperature plus swelling of the abdomen due to fluid accumulation that occurs as the dog's heart begins to fail. The final, critical stages include liver and kidney failure.

Discovery of most heartworm infestations is easily made by a veterinarian through use of a blood test that reveals the microfilariae. Occasionally, detection is more difficult if the worms are of only one sex or if they are older worms. Then, there may be no microfilariae present to be seen in a blood test. Many veterinarians offer a sophisticated blood test capable of detecting an antigen—a chemical change that occurs as the dog's body produces antibodies to the heartworm's presence. Once antibodies are detected, the veterinarian will likely recommend treatment unless the dog is in the advanced, most critical stages of the ailment.

Current therapy consists of a series of heartworm-killing, intravenous drug injections given to the dog during an overnight stay at the veterinarian's office. A follow-up treatment with a deworming product is done about a month later. Cost of the treatment is about $100, which is considered a bargain by owners whose dogs have been saved.

Once heartworm is well established in the dog, treatment can be more difficult, although it is successful in a majority of cases. The problem is that the adult heartworms are clustered in the dog's heart and arteries. Drugs are capable of killing these worms, but in doing their job they can damage the dog's liver, kidneys, or respiratory system. Another problem is that once the adult heartworms are dead, their remains float through the dog's bloodstream and can restrict blood flow. If the dog exercises during this period, it can suddenly die.

No dog should die from heartworms because prevention these days is so easy. Owners have their choice of pills that may be given in either daily or monthly doses.

Many Florida dog owners make the mistake of presuming that because they do not live near other dogs, or because their dog is kept inside, it cannot contract heartworms. However, every dog goes

Paramilitary dogs are purchased each year by the U.S. government for action in drugs and explosives detection and even as parachuting canine escorts for soldiers. Dogfaced recruits must be older than four years and weigh at least 50 pounds. Some may have to pass muster at the gun range by holding steady during pistol fire.

outside for walks, and infected mosquitoes may be carried for miles by breezes. Heartworm can infect any breed of dog at any age, and any responsible dog owner in Florida will see that the pet receives a heartworm preventative.

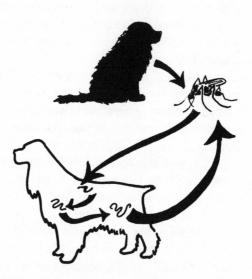

Heartworm starts when an infected dog is bitten by a mosquito. The infective larvae develop in the mosquito and are then deposited into another dog by a mosquito bite. The larvae develop and migrate to the dog's heart where they further develop and enter the bloodstream. The cycle continues after a mosquito bites the infected dog and spreads the disease to another host.

TAPEWORM

At some time or another, all Florida dogs are likely to have tapeworms, which are caused by the dog eating infected carrion or eating a flea that is in an infective stage.

The owner may notice sesame-seedlike objects in the dog's feces, on the tail end of the pet, or on the dog's bedding; these are segments from the tapeworm, which is living in the dog's gut. In time, the tapeworm will sap the nutrients from the dog's body, making the animal appear unkempt and underweight or suffer from diarrhea. Owners should be concerned because dog tapeworms can infect humans, although it is rare.

Ridding the dog of the worm is simple. After weighing the animal, a veterinarian will dispense a proper dose of dewormer, usually in tablet form. One dose of medication is generally sufficient to kill the tapeworm.

HOOKWORM

The hookworm is one of the most insidious dog killers. If undetected or left to grow unchecked, the small, comma-shaped worms suck blood and render the dog severely anemic.

The problem often begins when a hookworm-infected bitch delivers a litter of puppies. Hookworms are not transmitted to her puppies before birth, but through the mother's milk, particularly during the first week of the puppies' lives. The first symptom in an infected pup may be droopy behavior and an inability to gain weight. The owner may also notice that the dog has pale mucous membranes, an indication of anemia. Unfortunately, by the time the dog has reached such a serious stage of anemia, a veterinarian may not be able to save the dog.

Female dogs can be safely dewormed for hookworms from the fortieth day of pregnancy on and for two weeks after the puppies are born. The puppies should be dewormed for the first time when they are two weeks old.

Hookworm eggs pass from the dog's intestines to its living quarters through the feces. In typical Florida weather, the eggs hatch within seventy-two hours. The larval stage of the worm then contacts a dog's skin, burrows in, and searches for a convenient blood vessel to invade. The burrowing stage can produce intense itching, a signal to an astute owner that the pet has hookworms. Blood carries the worm through the lungs and eventually to the intestines. There, the parasite can live off the dog's blood, furnishing the world with more little hookworms.

In northern climates, the hookworm larvae are naturally killed by cold weather; in Florida, the larvae remain infective virtually all year.

Hookworms are pervasive Florida pests. One survey of dogs in Florida animal shelters found nearly 75 percent infected with hookworms. That same study found that even in dogs receiving routine veterinary care, the presence of hookworms was high, nearly 40 percent.

Dogs are not the only creatures who can be affected by hookworms. Children who play in areas where hookworm-infected dogs dirty the ground also are susceptible to infection. However, the canine hookworm does little more than make human skin itch intensely. It generally disappears after a few days.

ROUNDWORM

Unlike the hookworm, the large canine roundworm, *Toxocara canis*, can seriously afflict humans. The roundworm lives in the dog's intestines, producing hundreds of worm eggs each day. The worms then are passed from the dog's body to the soil, where they can be ingested by another dog or by a child playing in the area.

The Center for Disease Control in Atlanta reports that about 10,000 people contract roundworms each year. Of that number, nearly 1,000, usually children, suffer vision damage from the worm infestation. This occurs because the worm can penetrate the eye's retinal blood vessels.

Unfortunately, roundworm infestation may be difficult to notice. Many dog owners do not care to inspect dog vomit or feces where the worms may be observed.

Preventing roundworm infection in the household can be accomplished by regular deworming of the family pet and by insisting on good hygiene measures such as washing the hands before eating, especially after petting or playing with a dog. Children should not play in areas that dogs have used as a bathroom, and any dirty areas near the home should be cleaned regularly. No chemical has yet been discovered that can be sprayed on pet areas to kill roundworm larvae.

A pregnant dog can pass along the roundworm to her puppies. In fact, more than 90 percent of the roundworm transmissions occur before the puppies are born. About 5 percent of the roundworm infestations of puppies occur through the mother's milk. Wormy pups have pot bellies and straggly coats and usually suffer from diarrhea.

WHIPWORM

These worms can grow nearly three inches long in the dog's intestinal tract. Eggs are passed from the dog, and after fourteen to twenty-eight days on the warm, moist ground they become infective

Dogs are increasingly being used by exterminators to hunt down infestations of termites and carpenter ants. Beagles are a favorite breed for such work, but don't expect such canine expertise to come cheaply. The dog's termite evaluation costs about three times as much as traditional human inspection.

to other animals that may accidentally consume the larvae. Whipworm eggs can stay infective up to five years in a suitable environment. The usual signs of whipworm infection are weight loss, diarrhea, and, in severe cases, anemia.

DEWORMING

Control of nearly all the major canine worms is easily managed with dewormer chemicals available from veterinarians. Over-the-counter dewormers are dispensed for roundworms and hookworms, but it is wise to take the dog to a veterinarian before attempting to do the deworming yourself. The veterinarian will test the dog to determine the extent and nature of the infestation. Such a checkup also can reveal whether the dog is suffering from any severe side effects of worm infestation.

Veterinarians recommend that puppies be started on a deworming program at two weeks of age. Often, many of the canine worms can be eliminated with just one chemical. For instance, a heartworm preventative is available that also eliminates hookworms, roundworms, and whipworms. Dog owners should check with a veterinarian to determine the best type of dewormer and deworming routine for their own pets.

Unfortunately, worms are common in sunny Florida. If left unchecked to live inside the dog, these internal parasites always lead to health problems. Prevention is the key to avoiding such problems.

> *They say a reasonable number of fleas is good fer a dog—keeps him from broodin' over bein' a dog.*
> —Edward Noyes Westcott

CHAPTER 5

All Dogs Have Fleas

Hard-bodied, tenacious, 60-million-year-old blood suckers, fleas can become a major headache for the Florida dog and its owner. The state's year-round warm weather, particularly in the central and southern regions, is flea nirvana. In fact, the Tampa Bay area has been cited in a pesticide manufacturer's study as the second most flea-prone region in the United States. Similar studies reveal that October is the prime flea month for Florida dogs.

Basking in the warmth and humidity, fleas snuggle down into grass or carpeting to await the first passing warm-blooded animal—canine or human. They attach to a person's clothing, hitch a ride home, and then switch hosts, to dogs or other animals, where they feed on blood and lay eggs in the animal's fur.

FLEA LIFE CYCLE

Once in the house, adult fleas hop off Rover to lay eggs in carpeting, upholstery, or bedding. Still more eggs fall from the dog's fur. Depending on conditions, the flea eggs can hatch into tiny wrigglers within a few days. These larvae feed on household debris particles in carpeting or in floor crevices. Once mature, the larvae spin a cocoon and pupate for about five more days. In conditions that are properly warm, around 80 degrees, an adult flea will emerge to repeat the life cycle once more.

If a dog stays outdoors, an owner may not know to what extent fleas are sipping Fido's lifeblood. However, if the dog sleeps indoors, an owner soon will know fleas have taken up residence. A first clue is the owner's itching ankles.

Another telltale signal of flea infestation is the brown particles that can be seen anywhere the dog lies down. In the bath, this debris appears to wash off as blood. Actually, the flecks, which are flea feces deposited in the dog's fur, are composed of the dog's digested blood.

At this point, most dog owners declare war.

THE FLEA BATTLEGROUND

Armed with an arsenal of sprays, pills, flea collars, powders, dusts, dips, soaps, diatomaceous earth, and traps, the owner fires the first volleys of the "us or them" battle. But veterinarians caution that some of these "cures" may amount to proverbially shooting oneself in the foot. For example, some ingredients in flea cures can kill a dog, especially if several "cures" are used at the same time. Even shampoos and dips may cause a severe, even deadly, reaction if used in conjunction with the wrong types of flea collars, pills, or sprays.

One potentially dangerous ingredient is dichlorvos, also known as DDVP. Data accumulated by the National Institute of Health, the

> Veterinarians stress that flea eradication programs must include three areas: the dog (host), the house, and the yard or kennel. Spreadable granules containing Dursban are available from hardware or garden stores for the yard or kennel; products containing Dursban, Precor, or pyrethrin are effective in the house to prevent flea larvae from becoming adults; on the animal, pyrethrin-based products are advisable because of this chemical's minimal toxicity.

Environmental Protection Agency, and the Consumers Union suggest this chemical causes cancer in humans and dogs. DDVP may be regulated more stringently by the government in the future, but it currently is found in a range of flea-control products, so consumers should always check product labels.

Of course, too much of any pesticide used in the home can be risky. Children especially may develop an allergy or become sick after contact with an animal's flea collar or with an animal that has been recently bathed or dipped in a flea-control product. To be safe, dog owners should always check with their veterinarians about which pesticides are most effective and which ones may be combined with others.

Because dog owners have become more cautious about pesticide use, "natural" flea cures are appearing in advertisements and on the pet store shelves. One type is a "revolutionary" new flea control involving ultrasound, making the devices inaudible to humans and dogs. Manufacturers of these flea collars and boxes that can be placed in pet areas claim their products emit ultrasound waves. Fleas supposedly dislike ultrasound so much that they abandon the area.

The Environmental Protection Agency is not yet convinced that such gadgets actually repel fleas. The agency has ruled that ultrasound flea products may be marketed but must not claim to be effective on fleas. Research at the University of Florida's College of Veterinary Medicine failed to prove that one such device it tested was particularly repugnant to fleas.

Traps are another sort of pesticide-free flea cures. One type purports to attract fleas with a light, snaring them when they hop onto a sticky piece of paper near the light source. A variation of the sticky trap

> Statistics compiled by the University of Southern California's School of Medicine reveal:
> —Approximately 3 million dog bites occur annually in the U.S.
> —Boys over five years old are bitten by dogs twice as often as are girls.
> —Most bites occur in the summertime.
> —Three-fourths of the biting dogs are owned by the victim's neighbors.
> —Investigations reveal the victim antagonized the dog in most cases.
> —Most bites were of the hands or arms.

uses water. The claim is that the fleas drown in a pan of water once they're attracted by the light. Tests by entomologists with the U.S. Department of Agriculture found that some fleas did indeed hop into the water trap and die, but not in great enough numbers to make much difference in a flea-infested room.

Another unorthodox flea control is diatomaceous earth, composed of sharp skeletal particles from tiny marine algae. This very dusty repellent is used on the dog and the carpeting. Its intent is to kill not only fleas but other insects, such as roaches and ants, by slicing the insects' hard outer shells. Doing so causes death from moisture loss. It is effective, but messy.

Less effective is use of an amethyst crystal in a dog's water dish. Experts agree that fleas display no particular disdain for amethysts, and the dog could choke if it takes the crystal in its mouth.

Garlic, brewer's yeast, and B vitamins are also advertised as flea cure-alls, but tests have not proven any of them do much more than make the dog's skin and coat healthier. They have not been proven to repel fleas.

More promising, perhaps, is a product undergoing tests that comes out of Florida's famed citrus groves. It is made from orange peels. In early experiments, the peel's citrus oil has been found to kill fleas and, as a bonus, smells pleasant.

Yet another product, developed through a joint effort of the U.S. Department of Agriculture and the University of Florida's Institute of Food and Agriculture Sciences, promises to slow down the flea population. Preliminary findings say this product appears to control fleas indoors or outdoors for up to six months while being 90 percent effective and safer than most current pesticides. It works by inhibiting the growth of fleas, that is, by changing the flea's hormonal balance, and by preventing the development of the flea's hard outer shell.

In spite of the ever-increasing numbers of products, fleas continue to thrive, due in part to the flea's superior ability to develop immunity to pesticides. An insecticidal spray, shampoo, or dip that is used continuously becomes less effective as fleas develop resistance.

One fact on which entomologists and veterinarians agree is that fleas must be battled on three fronts: on the animal, in the yard (if it goes outside), and in the house. Dips and shampoos can be used to control fleas on the dog while sprays and foggers may be effective in

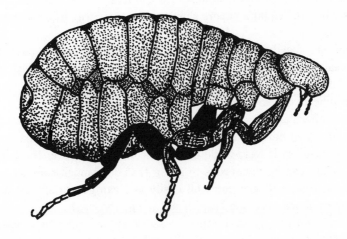

A close-up glimpse of Florida's primary canine pest. Fleas are active in the state nearly year-round. Once brought indoors, female fleas can lay hundreds of eggs in the household carpeting, the dog's coat, and the dog's bed. Within eight days, eggs hatch into white, wriggling larvae that spin cocoons within a week to a month. Fleas emerge from cocoons anytime from days to months depending on climate conditions and the availability of red-blooded hosts.

the yard and home, but owners are again cautioned to use only controls that can be applied simultaneously without producing a chemically toxic by-product. In the home, the contents of foggers tend to coat furniture, bedding, and even food with a chemical residue. Foggers should be used judiciously in homes with infants or young children.

Flea collars, like foggers, are a popular flea control. The idea behind such collars is that they kill fleas by emitting chemical vapors that supposedly spread throughout the dog's coat. Many dogs despise flea collars and must be hog-tied when a new collar is fastened around their necks. If the collar is taken from its container and allowed to air out for a day, dogs do not seem to object as much to the pungent vapors. Still, many canine Houdinis will occupy themselves for days, if necessary, working to escape from a flea collar.

Flea collars are not among the veterinary world's favorite flea-battling devices for several reasons. One is that the collars have virtually no "knock-down" effect. That means the collars do not prompt a mass flea evacuation from the dog. Rover still suffers the fleas while the collar's vapors slowly make their way into the animal's fur.

Another disadvantage cited by veterinarians is that many dogs, especially light-colored or white dogs, may suffer severe lesions on their necks from the collars. These may be simple allergies, or they may indicate a toxic reaction to the collar's chemicals.

Then there are the special problems of flea collars on dogs used for hunting or other outdoor activities. Some brands of flea collars become useless if wet, while others become more toxic. In addition, flea collars can be dangerous to a dog that does much running; some types of collars do not come off easily and can get caught on a tree stump or fence post and trap, if not hang, the dog.

Many veterinarians advise that the safest and most effective household flea control at the dog owner's disposal is the simplest—the vacuum cleaner. Fleas at all stages of development can be sucked up in any properly operating vacuum. Thorough flea control may necessitate daily suctioning of either the dog or the carpeting, or both. Following a vacuuming, the cleaner bag should be either immediately disposed

> The Center for Disease Control in Atlanta reports that at least 157 people in the U.S. died from dog attacks during the past ten years, and more than 40 percent of the deaths were attributed to pit bulldogs.

of or sprayed with a shot of an insecticide to keep the fleas from escaping and reinfesting the home or pet area.

Rug shampooing a couple of times during the summer also decreases household flea populations. Even such a simple measure as routinely washing pet bedding can help keep the flea problem at bay.

FLEA-CAUSED PROBLEMS

Danger of flea-carried disease is not usually a problem. It was the rat flea, not the dog flea, that transmitted the bubonic plague during the Middle Ages.

However, fleas do cost dog owners money. Most of it is spent to control the pests, but other costs arise as fleas irritate the dog, causing it to chew on itself. So-called hot spots can become infected. Tapeworms also may appear when dogs inadvertently consume an infective flea.

> **"** *If you pick up a starving dog and make him prosperous, he will not bite you. This is the principal difference between a dog and a man.*
> *—Mark Twain* **"**

CHAPTER **6**

Fur Is Only Skin Deep

A perpetual sun with its constant warming rays continues to attract people, and their dogs, to the Sunshine State. For people, such climatic conditions evoke a sense of well-being, but for their dogs, these same subtropical conditions often bring on a variety of skin problems, many of which can prompt Fido to chew himself until he draws blood.

ALLERGIES

Immune responses to a wide variety of substances are part of a normal dog's bodily protection system. Anything such as food, plant pollen, fungi, drugs, microbes, dust, insects, chemicals—even sunshine, can prompt the immune system to react.

If a dog is ultrasensitive to such substances, the response may be a negative reaction that is known as an allergy. In an allergic dog, the immune system malfunctions and the animal's body produces chemicals that cause tissue damage, which causes further injurious immune responses.

Exactly why one dog has an allergic response to fleas, for instance, while another dog does not, remains an area for research. One theory holds that some dogs have a genetic tendency, or susceptibility, toward allergic reactions called atopy.

Allergic responses can range from a runny nose or eyes to intense itching, breathing difficulties, or vomiting and diarrhea. In extreme instances, a dog can go into shock.

If the dog exhibits allergic symptoms, it is advisable to seek help from a veterinarian. Some allergies can be alleviated with desensitization treatments in which the dog is injected with tiny portions of the allergy-causing agent. Slowly, the dog's immune system begins to respond properly. In other situations, little can be done except to keep the dog away from known allergens and to treat the animal with symptom-easing drugs.

Flea Allergy

A common irritation of the Florida dog's skin is caused by biting fleas. But diagnosing the problem can be tricky because it may not be the individual flea bites that are the irritant but, instead, an allergy resulting from the flea bites. If the skin eruptions disappear once the dog is flea-free, it's a good bet the dog has an allergy to the bites.

Research at the University of Florida revealed that more can be better when it comes to fleas. Household pets that were rarely exposed to fleas were found to develop allergies more readily once they were exposed to fleas. That's because flea bites produce antigens, an irritant that can trigger allergies. The University of Florida study found that dogs seldom bitten by fleas responded more severely to the flea antigen and more often developed an allergic reaction. On the other hand, the same study found that dogs such as animal shelter strays who were constantly exposed to fleas tended to develop a tolerance to flea antigen and suffered fewer and less severe allergic reactions.

There is no cure for flea allergy. Symptoms can be somewhat controlled with corticosteroids, but these can cause side effects such as weight gain and kidney problems. Results of current research seem to indicate that occasional flea bites actually may keep a dog from developing the allergic reaction.

Miscellaneous Allergies

Another cause of itchy Fidos is as simple as a dog bath: the too-frequently-shampooed dog may be allergic to the soap or may be suffering from dry skin.

Flea-control products also may produce irritation or allergic reactions in some dogs, but that is more difficult to track down. Improvement may be achieved by changing to a product with different chemicals in it. Veterinarians may opt to take skin tests to pinpoint the source of a dog's itching.

As for the dog with flea allergy dermatitis, control of any allergic reactions may require use of cortisone products to keep the dog comfortable through the most severe bouts of itching.

MANGE

Mange is caused by mites, which may be either the sarcoptic type or the demodectic type. These two types of mites, both prevalent in Florida, have their own peculiar habits. The sarcoptic mange mite makes burrows in the skin; the demodectic mite enters hair follicles and oil glands in the skin.

Sarcoptic mange causes intense itching as the mite buries itself in the dog's skin. The skin dries, thickens, and wrinkles, and crusts form, usually around the dog's eyes, ears, and mouth. Mange then spreads to the neck, legs, tail, and abdomen of the dog. Persons handling a dog diagnosed with this type of mange should use gloves and minimize contact because *Sarcoptes* mites will infect humans.

In demodectic infestations, the dog's skin lesions may vary from red running sores to small hairless patches. In severe cases, the mites may invade the dog's lymph nodes.

Presence of either type of mange can be determined by a skin scraping. Once the mange is properly diagnosed, a veterinarian can recommend the best wash or dip to end the scourge. It generally takes several treatments. Clipping the affected dog's coat, especially if it is long, is normal procedure.

Demodectic mange is the more difficult type to cure and requires patience on the part of the owner, who may have to massage medication into the dog's skin for a month or more. Secondary infection can occur from mange and that may have to be treated with antibiotics. Home remedies for demodectic mange are not advisable. They are ineffective and can delay treatment, allowing the condition to grow worse.

MISCELLANEOUS SKIN PROBLEMS

Occasionally, nutritional deficiencies, hormonal imbalances, bee or wasp stings, skin tumors, diabetes—even sunlight or grass allergies—can prompt some dogs' skin to swell or become inflamed.

Dachshunds can become affected by an ailment known as *Acanthosis nigricans*. It is believed that glandular malfunctioning may play a role in producing raw spots, crusts, and patches of thickened skin. Often the lesions appear wherever the dog rubs its skin on a hard surface. In severe instances, this itchy and oozing skin disease covers the dog from its ears to its abdomen. Secondary infection is of particular concern. While the condition can be controlled by veterinarians, no permanent cure has been reported.

German shepherds, Shetland sheepdogs, and mixes of these two breeds can suffer a facial eczema. The bridge of the nose is usually the first area to show symptoms of bleeding and crusting. Keeping the dog out of Florida's intense sun and applying lotion with sun screen can help prevent the problem.

Treatment of these more obscure skin problems requires specific diagnosis by a veterinarian. But one procedure that has been helpful is desensitizing shots. In the case of bee sting allergies, dogs have been injected with the insect venom and have successfully overcome the allergy.

Ohio State University studies found that another skin ailment, ideopathic seborrheic dermatitis, may be related to the way a dog's skin grows. This dermatitis is a foul-smelling, excessively scaly condition that occurs with no known cause. Dogs with seborrhea suffer with inflamed, oily, thickened skin that generally requires veterinary treatment. The condition often abates but then recurs. The study revealed that grafting normal skin onto the affected areas vastly improves the ailment in laboratory animals. Researchers believe this procedure worked because the grafted skin slowed down the abnormally fast growth of the top layer of seborrheic skin. Studies are still underway so grafting may not be available to dog owners until some future date.

RINGWORM
This fungal condition often makes not only the dog's life miserable but the owner's as well. Humans contract the itchy condition that is characterized by a semicircular-shaped brown crust.

Ringworm is wildly contagious. Once it gets started in a kennel, it can infect the skin of every canine resident. Fortunately, it often cures itself in about six weeks; not so fortunately, some cases of ringworm are tough to cure.

Most ringworm fungi are easily dispatched with an antifungal cream from the veterinarian. An oral treatment also is available, but it is expensive and some owners have reported side effects in their dogs such as vomiting.

Colorado researchers report that a new process using hot radio waves is quite successful in treating ringworm. An electrode heated to about 122 degrees is applied to the affected area and kills the fungus without burning the skin. This method is still in the experimental stages but promises a bright future in treating ringworm and in the removal of warts, cysts, and tumors. Some scarring of delicate areas has been reported.

TICKS
City dogs enjoy a relatively tick-free existence, but because Florida is a paradise of year-round flora, the state's dog owners should always be alert to these blood-sucking parasites. Country dogs, especially those used in hunting or taken along on camping trips, are most

prone to tick infestation. Ticks hide on leaves and crawl upon available hosts, be they dog or human.

The *common dog tick* is a scourge to canines all year in Florida, but it is most prevalent from April through September, with June as a peak month. Adults are reddish-brown. The *Gulf Coast tick* frequents coastal areas of Florida. Adults are dark brown with silvery lines and spots and tend to attach to a dog's ears.

Dogs that have been in the woods should always be inspected for ticks. One or two ticks is tolerable to a dog, but often the site of a single tick bite can become irritated and infected. In large numbers, ticks will cause anemia, weight loss, and even paralysis.

Tick Paralysis

Tick paralysis most often afflicts hunting dogs, but any dog may be susceptible. The paralysis is believed to be caused by a nerve-killing toxin produced by ticks when they feed on the blood of their host.

First sign of the paralysis is generally a loss of coordination in the dog's hindquarters. The animal may not be able to walk steadily. Reflexes then slow over a period of a couple of days and the dog may become totally immobilized, yet retain a bright look and appetite. The effects of tick paralysis can disappear within hours after removal of the parasites, though severe cases may take a week to recover. In some cases, the paralysis may affect breathing and cause death.

Clearly, any paralysis of a dog would suggest a visit to the veterinarian.

Rocky Mountain Spotted Fever

Florida veterinarians report an increasing number of dogs with Rocky Mountain spotted fever. Fortunately, the disease is usually mild, with appetite loss and fever as common symptoms. Further danger from the tick that carries this disease arises to the dog's owner. Dogs can bring the fever tick into the house, where it can infect humans.

Lyme Disease

A disease among dogs and humans was noticed in Old Lyme, Connecticut, some years back. It now has spread to the South. A certain tick-borne bacteria produces fever, loss of appetite, swollen lymph glands, and arthritis in dogs or their owners. Unfortunately, early symptoms are subtle and it takes an astute veterinarian to promptly diagnose Lyme disease.

Treatment with antibiotics brings about relief from symptoms, although it is not 100 percent effective.

Tick Infestation

Signs of tick infestation include head shaking, scratching, loss of appetite, even tearing. The most common sites are the dog's head, ears, neck, flanks, and between its toes.

The method of removing ticks depends on the numbers infesting the dog. A few ticks can be tweezed off with a dab of kerosene on a tissue. Care should be taken to make sure the tick's mouth parts are not left attached to the skin.

Veterinarians now report that tick-borne diseases such as Rocky Mountain spotted fever and Lyme disease can be contracted by people who use their bare hands to remove ticks from their dogs. Tick feces, crushed body parts, or fluid can transmit disease through an owner's skin, even though there are no evident skin cuts or abrasions. Always wear gloves and use tweezers to remove ticks.

Dipping the dog in a tick-killing compound is a sure way to ensure all ticks are removed from the outside of the dog. The inside of the dog's ears should be checked and wiped with a mild solution of the chemical. As with flea-control products, tick pesticides can be toxic if not used in proper strength or if mixed with other chemicals. Veterinarians can recommend the most effective and safest chemical.

EAR MITES

A tiny, waxy-colored parasitic mite lives on the surface of the skin near many dogs' ears. It feeds in and around the ear and may proceed into the ear canal.

In south Florida especially, the mites plague dogs year-round. In central and north Florida, where occasional freezes contain the mite population, dogs are slightly less affected.

Dogs with ear mites shake their heads and rub their ears with their

> A biting dog exerts from 150 to 200 pounds of pressure per square inch of jaw power. Trained guard dogs can bite more than twice that hard.

paws, rub against furniture, and may come repeatedly to their owners to have their ears massaged.

Owners can recognize the presence of mites by a brown scum that coats the ear region. Drops of mineral oil or an oily product made specifically for ear mites will loosen and kill the mites. The ear should be gently massaged after the oil is applied. A wire loop may be used to gently clean around the ear. Swabs are not recommended because they may pack the dirty material back into the ear. Repeating the ear-oiling every three days may be necessary.

Some veterinarians recommend washing out the ear mites with a mild mix of warm water and lotion-type dishwashing soap (not dishwashing machine soap). The mix should be about a quarter teaspoon of soap to one cup of water. With a medicine dropper, the mixture can be squeezed into the dog's ear and massaged. The dog then shakes its ears and the dirt is flung out. The ear should be dried with a soft towel. The procedure may be continued until the ear looks clean.

Both treatments eliminate not only the adult ear mites but the up-and-comers as well.

If ear mites are ignored, which is sometimes difficult with persistently itching dogs, the ear can form cystlike pools of blood known as hematomas. Dogs with drooping ears are the most usual victims. Ear mites are believed to contribute to hematomas by prompting the dog to shake its head. One treatment reduces the hematoma with a needle. But some veterinarians report that this procedure can result in recurrence of the problem. Better results are reported with a surgery to remove the hematoma. Some animals have to be sedated following treatment to prevent head shaking while the surgery heals.

> **❝***He stood with his muzzle thrust out through the door The whole forty days of that terrible pour! Because of which drenching, the Sages unfold, The nose of a healthy dog is always cold.***❞**
> *—Arthur Guiterman*

CHAPTER 7

Unchained Maladies

Florida statute 585.195 lists five canine diseases against which dogs that are sold must be vaccinated: distemper, hepatitis, leptospirosis, tracheobronchitis, and canine parvovirus. At first glance, it appears that a most serious contagious disease—canine rabies—has been omitted. However, the statute also states that any dog sold must have a health certificate that states the animal is free of contagious disease, and that includes rabies, albeit subtly. As a rule of thumb, to cover all eventualities Florida dogs should receive annual inoculation for all of these diseases.

The initial symptoms of all these ailments is fever, plus altered behavior such as listlessness or irritability.

RABIES

Perhaps the most well-known, and feared, viral canine disease is largely preventable by vaccination.

Transmission of rabies to unprotected dogs can come from many sources: other dogs or cats, or by contact with virtually any warm-blooded animal including cattle or horses. The virus is generally transmitted through a bite, when an uninfected dog is bitten by a rabies-infected animal. The virus can be carried in the saliva of an infected animal for days before the typical symptoms appear.

Rabies affects the animal's central nervous system in two phases. The first, which the medical world defines as "prodromal," means the initial phase of the onset of disease. It lasts from one to three days, during which the animal's behavior changes slightly. It may stop eating and drinking and may seek to sleep in a dark corner.

The second phase may take the "mad dog" form, in which the infected dog exhibits extreme irritability and will bite at any provocation. Light and noise produce excitability because the animal's senses are overly sensitized by the virus. An owner of a rabies-vicious dog may notice that it eats strange objects such as stones. An affected dog will chew or bite at anything. The inevitable outcome, within ten days, is the animal's death.

Not all rabid dogs exhibit viciousness. The second rabies phase may manifest itself as paralysis. In these instances, the dog is unable to control its jaws or its salivation, and after a few hours, the virus affects an increasing number of muscles. Without ever turning particularly vicious, the dog simply lapses into a coma and dies.

Rabies are transmissible to humans during both phases—either through the bite of a vicious "mad" dog or through the large quantities of saliva produced by the paralytic dog. Indeed, paralytic rabies may be more dangerous than vicious rabies to dog owners or handlers. Traditionally, rabies has been stereotyped as a disease of "mad" dogs

Each year approximately 200 cases of rabies-infected animals are reported in Florida. Most are wild animals, but some are pets. Any dog sold in Florida must have a health certificate and have received a rabies vaccination. On top of that, counties and municipalities may have their own requirements. All dogs in Florida, whether they wander outdoors or remain indoors, should be vaccinated for rabies.

who froth at the mouth. Thus, the owner whose dog is simply drooling or suffering paralysis may not take proper precautions and may come in contact with the dog's virus-infected saliva.

Rabies virus is harbored in the affected dog's saliva. Any dog that exhibits the symptoms of either vicious or paralytic rabies should be gingerly handled with gloved hands or a dogcatcher's loop. The dog should be confined as quickly as possible to minimize its contact with people or other animals.

Confinement is mandatory for suspected rabies carriers. In the case of human exposure, the animal likely will be killed to relieve its suffering and its brain will be examined for presence of rabies virus. There have been instances where an animal was killed and then was found not to be rabid. Animal scientists are working to develop a test for rabies that does not depend on examining the dead animal's brain tissues.

Exposed humans are advised to take the five-shot "post-exposure" rabies injections to prevent contracting the disease. The shots are no longer given in the stomach but in the arm and are much improved over the formerly "painful" rabies shots.

The diligence of Florida health officials has ensured that human deaths due to rabies are practically nonexistent. No Floridian has died from rabies since 1948. Still, anyone in the business of breeding or showing dogs should receive pre-exposure immunization, and all dogs should be reimmunized every year for peak protection.

Rabies Incidence in Florida's Animals

Florida's confirmed animal rabies cases between 1978 and 1987 have varied from 47 cases in 1978 to a high of 183 cases in 1986.

Statistics from the state Department of Health reveal that Floridians, or their dogs, are most likely to contract rabies if they come in contact with raccoons. Since 1978, confirmed rabies has occurred in the following animals:

Animal	Number
raccoons	770
bats	256
foxes	44
cats	33
dogs	22
skunks	20
bobcats	10
horses	5
cattle	2
otters	2
opossums	1

But wildlife experts warn that conclusions drawn from the above statistics can be misleading. The likelihood of coming in contact with such statistically-high rabies animals as raccoons or bats is much lower than coming in contact with cats or dogs.

State statistics indicate that the highest numbers of confirmed rabies cases occur in such populous counties as those listed below. But ironically, the fewest confirmed cases list includes the state's most densely populated county, Pinellas. Likewise, populous Dade County has had just four confirmed rabies cases between 1978 and 1987. Thus, attempting to determine whether there is a lesser incidence of rabies in urban or rural locales is inconclusive.

Top Five Animal Rabies Counties, 1978–87

County	Total Confirmed Cases
Polk	109
Leon	99
Duval	78
Orange	69
Escambia	49

Counties with Fewest Confirmed Animal Rabies Cases, 1978–87

Hendry	0
Pinellas	0
Monroe	0
Sumter	0
Union	0
Dixie	1
Glades	1
Liberty	1

Many owners self-administer rabies immunization vaccine to their dogs. Though it may be more economical and more convenient than visiting the veterinarian, it is against state law for an owner to immunize a dog for a disease that is transmissible to humans. Florida law specifies that only veterinarians may immunize animals for four specific diseases, of which one is rabies. (The other three are brucellosis, tuberculosis, and equine encephalomyelitis.)

DISTEMPER

Caused by a highly contagious virus related to measles, distemper is spread through the air or by contaminated objects. Initial symptoms are subtle and may not be noticed by an owner until two or three weeks after the dog has been exposed.

The first observable symptom is a brief fever, lasting only a few days. A second fever, lasting about a week, may then occur. At this time the owner may notice a discharge from the dog's eyes, which are reddened. The dog may squint at bright light. A depressed appetite and diarrhea develop. Some dogs display lameness, refusing to walk on one or more of their legs ("hardpad" disease). In some cases, dogs

Veterinarians at Auburn University have developed a dog hearing aid. They found, after surveying hundreds of small animal practices, that many dogs suffer hearing losses. The drawbacks: The hearing aids are scarce and available from just a few medical centers, and many dogs cannot be trained to wear the aids.

appear to improve only to develop later symptoms such as muscle twitching, followed by paralysis of the hindquarters and convulsions.

Veterinarians recommend first vaccinating puppies for distemper by age eight weeks, followed by a second vaccination at three or four months. An annual distemper vaccination is strongly recommended. Many adult dog distemper cases seen by veterinarians occur needlessly because owners do not know that distemper vaccinations should be given annually.

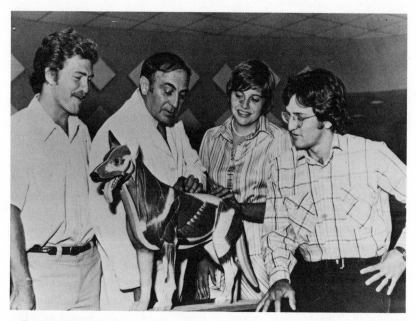

Students at the University of Florida's College of Veterinary Medicine must master basic canine anatomy.

HEPATITIS

Infectious canine hepatitis (ICH) affects dogs of all ages. The virus is usually transmitted by severely ill animals via all bodily secretions, although a rare respiratory form of the illness can be spread through the air. The incubation period after exposure is from five to nine days.

The initial symptom is a fever of about 104 degrees (normal temperature is 100–102 degrees) that lasts from one to six days.

Other symptoms include listlessness, loss of appetite, thirst, reddened eyes that are excessively weepy, nasal discharge, vomiting, and, occasionally, bruising and soreness of the abdomen accompanied by swelling of the head, neck, and body.

A key to diagnosing ICH is having the dog's blood checked by a veterinarian for reduced clotting time. Although ICH symptoms can closely mimic those of distemper, positive diagnosis usually is made by testing tissue samples from the dog's liver.

LEPTOSPIROSIS

A disease that affects dogs of any age, leptospirosis will affect male dogs more often than females dogs. Incubation of this disease is from five to fifteen days after exposure.

Initial symptoms can appear rapidly and include slight weakness, appetite loss, vomiting, a temperature of from 103 degrees to 105 degrees, and mild reddening of the eyes. Diagnosis at this stage of the ailment can be difficult because leptospirosis resembles other diseases.

Within two days of the initial symptoms, however, leptospirosis prompts a sudden drop in temperature, pronounced depression of the animal, labored breathing, and insatiable thirst. The animal will hesitate to get up or do anything that uses the hind legs, and may exhibit pain in the hind area. If the owner checks the dog's mouth, burnlike abrasions may be apparent and the animal may have difficulty swallowing. Advanced cases produce muscle tremors and a temperature decline as low as 97 degrees.

Although leptospirosis symptoms appear frightening, veterinarians report that rarely more than 10 percent of the infected dogs die. Antibiotic treatment is generally effective.

This is a disease that can occur in "epidemics." Owners should maintain contact with their veterinarians, and if an outbreak is noted

---

Dogs can catch diseases from their owners. One of the most common man-to-dog illnesses is strep throat.

by the medical community, vaccination may be required more frequently than once a year.

PARVOVIRUS

Although dogs of all ages may contract this disease, puppies are most susceptible. Parvo, as it is called, is nothing to trifle with. It is a gastrointestinal virus, discovered in 1978, that spread throughout the world before science developed a vaccine.

Symptoms include listlessness, bloody diarrhea, vomiting, and dehydration. The dog's abdomen may be sore when touched. Body temperature of adult dogs with parvo may be normal, but in puppies it is more likely to be as high as 106 degrees. Unfortunately, many of the symptoms of parvo closely resemble ICH, but a veterinarian can take tests to positively identify the virus.

If prompt treatment is given, dogs can fully recover from this disease. Veterinarians stress that parvo causes much suffering and death, yet the current vaccines are effective. An annual parvo vaccination renders this disease highly preventable.

INFECTIOUS TRACHEOBRONCHITIS

This relatively mild ailment is dubbed "kennel cough" because it is highly contagious and can spread posthaste through a kennel. Dogs of any age can be infected.

The incubation of this virus is generally five to ten days. The most noticeable symptom is a dreadfully husky cough that can occur in spasms, especially after the dog has exercised. It is not unusual for a dog to throw up or gag during coughing spells. Infection is usually limited to the animal's windpipe and bronchi. The worst stage passes within five days, but kennel cough can continue in a less severe form for up to twenty days. If the problem persists, a secondary bacterial infection may have invaded the dog. Dogs that are kept in poor conditions may have recurring bouts of this virus. Fortunately, veterinary treatment generally remedies kennel cough within days.

CORONAVIRAL GASTROENTERITIS

In 1978, this relatively rare but highly contagious disease appeared in some show dogs. The primary symptoms are vomiting, diarrhea,

> Research reveals some dog breeds are more prone to heart problems due to the deficient production of carnitine. Boxers, Doberman pinschers, and St. Bernards are most often afflicted. Injections of carnitine have reportedly helped dogs that suffer from lack of oxygen due to a poorly performing heart.

and appetite loss that may appear suddenly in an apparently healthy animal. Puppies stricken with coronavirus can die quickly, usually from dehydration.

Veterinarians in rural areas do not report many cases of coronavirus, but urban veterinarians are including this disease in their routine vaccine schedule. Kennel owners should be especially wary of this disease because of its contagiousness.

> *He is gentle, he is kind. I'll never, never find a better friend than old dog Tray.*
> —*Stephen Foster*

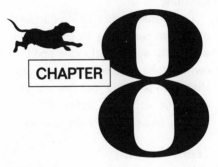

CHAPTER

8

Bumps in the Florida Night

F lorida's environment can be an enjoyable haven for pet owners, but for dogs the state's unique climate promotes an array of potentially troublesome insects and plant life as well as environmental hazards that may not occur anywhere else in the United States.

Keeping dogs safe from Florida's unique hazards is not difficult.

> A common myth is that a dog heals itself by licking a wound. In fact, a dog's constant licking can inflame or even infect a wound.

Awareness of the dangers, most of which are seldom encountered by the average dog, is the best way to prevent dog injuries or fatalities. (You'll also find some helpful first-aid procedures in Chapter 9.)

WEATHER

Florida is dubbed "The Sunshine State" for a very good reason: the sun shines here nearly 70 percent of the time. Even winter days are warmed to an average of 64 degrees by what seems to be eternal sunshine.

Temperatures in Florida during the hottest months reach 90 degrees along the coastlines to the mid-90s in the interior of the state. This abundant solar bath can spell serious problems for dogs. While owners take refuge from the steamy air, they often assume erroneously that Fido is faring just fine out in the back yard without a pinpoint of shade or sufficient water. That is not the case. Dogs suffer, as do people, from heat stroke and sunburn.

Heat Stroke

Many heat stroke cases are caused by leaving a dog enclosed in a car. Temperatures inside a car on a typical 85-degree Florida day, even with the windows open slightly, will reach 102 degrees within ten minutes. After the panting animal has been in the closed car for a half-hour, the temperature inside the vehicle is close to 120 degrees.

A dog does not produce sweat via pores over his body; instead, he cools his body temperature primarily by panting. In temperatures of 120-plus degrees, however, the dog's body temperature can rise to a fatal 108 degrees as the heat of the car is too much for the dog's cooling system to handle. Too many unthinking dog owners have returned to their cars only to find their pet convulsing or already dead.

It is against Florida's cruelty to animals statute to leave a dog unattended inside an automobile. Offenders can be charged with animal cruelty and fined up to $5,000.

But not all heat stroke occurs because animals are left in cars. Any dog that is confined to an unshaded area may build up an internal body temperature beyond which its body can cope. Puppies and older dogs are especially susceptible to Florida's solar rays.

Thunder and Lightning

Florida dogs frequently develop a keen fear of thunder and crawl under the bed or to a secluded spot at the first peal of a storm. Such a reaction is understandable considering the violence of Florida storms, which can be fearsome even to a native Floridian or old-timer. As newcomers soon learn, the state is one of the nation's prime thunderstorm regions, due to the abundant heat and humidity. Statistics compiled by the National Weather Service reveal that each year Florida has an average of 120 days in which thunderstorms occur.

There is not much an owner can do to calm a storm-frightened dog until the noise moves on. Most dogs do settle down once they are secure in their hiding places, but in severe instances, dogs that have been left alone, especially if their regular storm bunkers are closed off, have suffered heart attacks during thunderstorms.

Owners who leave their pets alone during the state's prime thunderstorm months—May until August—should consider providing their pets with a place to hunker down during a storm. Indoors, if the dog does not have his own bed, a bathroom or a hall closet can provide Fido with peace of mind. A small table or even a piano bench can serve as refuge when temporarily covered by an old sheet or drop cloth. Outside dogs should have a secure shelter in which to wait out nature's noisy fireworks. A dog that is obviously terrorized by loud thunder can be given a prescription pet tranquilizer prior to storms.

Lightning can kill dogs if they are in a precarious outside location during a storm. Outdoor dogs should never be tied to a tree or leashed to a wire exercise runner during a lightning storm.

In Florida's northern counties, thunderstorms are not as severe as they are in the state's central and southern areas. Similarly, temperatures in north Florida are milder during summer but cooler in winter—cold enough at times for snow to fall, particularly in the Panhandle. Dogs should be provided shelter in cold weather, but even the coolest

Florida nights seldom prove life-threatening to dogs as long as they have an enclosure to block the north winds.

Other threats of nature, although rarely encountered by the average urban dog owner in Florida, do exist throughout the state. Snakes, alligators, a multitude of insects, poisonous plants, and marine hazards such as jellyfish are always at the ready to surprise the unwitting or careless dog owner.

POISONOUS SNAKES

Eastern Diamondback Rattlesnake

Florida has its share of pit vipers. The eastern diamondback rattlesnake, a Florida native, is the largest and can be found in all of the state's sixty-seven counties and on coastal islands. Its most likely habitat is in palmetto scrub, abandoned fields, and pine woods, all of which provide perfect cover for rattlers. Their familiar diamond pattern of browns and beiges makes them difficult to spot.

While some snakebites occur because a dog steps on a snake or leaps over a log onto a rattler, veterinarians report that most snake-bitten dogs they treat have facial wounds. This can occur when the curious dog barks or taunts the snake. Under normal circumstances, if a rattlesnake is given an opportunity, it will retreat and hide. If a dog and rattlesnake face off, the snake generally will coil and strike at the intruder. Striking capability is a distance of about one-third to one-half the snake's body length.

Two myths prevail about rattlesnakes: they always strike from a coiled position, and they always rattle their tail to warn of an impending strike. In fact, rattlers have been known to strike when not coiled, and they often will strike without sounding their rattle.

If struck by a rattlesnake, many dogs will survive if the owner can get the dog to an antivenin source quickly (see also Chapter 9).

Canebrake Rattlesnake

This snake is found primarily in north Florida, rarely seen farther south than the Gainesville area. It is less commonly encountered than the diamondback, so most people don't recognize the canebrake when they see it.

The canebrake has a gray-brown or pinkish color with dark bands across its body and an orange or rust-colored stripe down the middle of its back. It is more slender than the diamondback variety. Like its larger cousin, the canebrake is also found in abandoned fields, but it also may seek watering holes in swampy areas during the hot months of the year.

Pygmy Rattlesnake

Found throughout Florida, these tiny (less than eighteen inches long) stout-bodied gray snakes are quick to strike. The pygmy's favorite hiding spots include palmetto scrub, pine woods, and ponds or marshes.

This small snake rarely produces a bite that is life-threatening to a dog. The bite is painful, however, and should be checked by a veterinarian.

Cottonmouth (Water Moccasin)

No noise warns intruders of the presence of this silently gliding, sometimes aggressive water snake. Florida cottonmouths are usually about three feet long and can be found in virtually any of the state's freshwater regions—from the smallest creek to the largest pond or lake.

Cottonmouths do provide a vague warning of a strike by offering a silently gaping yawn that reveals a dazzlingly white mouth. From a loose coil or uncoiled, and from dry land or in the water, this snake's strike is breathtakingly fast. It hunts primarily at night and spends its days in more sluggish pursuits such as sunbathing.

This snake's bite can be as serious as that of a rattlesnake if not attended to quickly.

Coral Snake

A colorful relative of the cobra, the krait, and the mamba, the Florida coral snake is the most poisonous of all, especially for its small size, which is only about two feet long. Fortunately, it is a shy and secretive creature that bothers only the most curious dogs (or owners) who insist on poking about woodpiles or in deep piles of fallen leaves.

Coral snakes are frequently confused with the harmless scarlet king snake. Both have alternating bands of red, black, and yellow. Admittedly, most people fail to hang around long enough to discover the differences between the two snake species. But if they did, they would see that the scarlet king snake has a red nose, while the coral snake's nose is black. Or, this simple rhyme can be memorized: "Red touch yellow, kill a fellow; red touch black, good for Jack." That means the coral snake's red and yellow bands touch each other, while the scarlet king's red and black rings touch.

Coral snakes do not strike. Rather, they chew their victim, injecting a deadly venom with each chomp. A dog is in greatest danger if the snake gets attached to the pup's nose and is reluctant to let go. However, reported dog fatalities from coral snake bites are rare.

ALLIGATORS

Once hunted nearly to extinction, Florida's official state reptile has made a stunning comeback, and the state's alligator population is now estimated at about one million. That number prompts phone calls every day to game and law enforcement officials reporting some errant alligator that has found its way onto a driveway or lawn or into someone's private pond or swimming pool.

Most alligators are willing to live quietly alongside humans. But once fed by people, the alligator often becomes a dangerous nuisance. The reptiles become accustomed to a handout and (never known for astounding intelligence) can grow not just hungry, but angry if the treat is withheld. And that's when they become dangerous to dogs and people.

Many Florida visitors and transplanted residents don't realize that the usually lumbering alligator, if riled or searching for food, can prop itself up on its little lizard legs and race with startling agility toward prey on land. Some wildlife rangers report clocking a frenzied alligator at a speed close to that of a quarter horse. Moreover, alligators can climb fences, launching themselves with their sturdy tails up and over an obstacle.

If a particular waterway contains a breeding pair of alligators, the duo can become nuisances during the summer mating season after the female has laid her eggs. She will be highly protective of her nest and likely will challenge any dog that wanders too near.

Dogs may survive an alligator attack, but more usually the small breeds are seized and dragged into the water, where the reptile will finish its meal.

Preventing such a horror is the dog owner's best solution. Here are a few tips to keep dogs safe from alligator jaws:

—*Never* feed an alligator.

—Keep watch on any alligator in nearby waterways. If one begins showing aggressive tendencies, such as starting to chase after people or animals, call the local Florida Game and Fresh Water Fish Commission office. The agency can relocate the reptile. Never attempt to capture a nuisance alligator yourself.

—Do not allow a dog to wander unattended near waterways known to contain alligators.

POISONOUS TOADS

A deadly threat to Florida dogs, particularly those that live in south Florida, is the poisonous giant toad (*Bufo marinus*). No ordinary specimen, this brown toad is immense—up to seven inches long. It

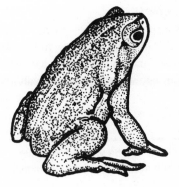

Sometimes growing as large as seven inches, the giant toad *(Bufo marinus)* can poison dogs. Its size is an immediate identifier, but the swollen glands above the front legs also mark this poisonous amphibian.

has two large poison sacs called paratoid glands that extend downward from the head to the rib cage.

Curious dogs that play with and mouth this toad can die if they consume enough of the paratoid-secreted toxin. Some studies have indicated nearly a 100 percent mortality rate among Florida dogs who have ingested the poison.

The first symptoms of toad poisoning can be as subtle as excessive salivation or as dramatic as convulsive seizures, depending on the age and health of the affected dog. Death usually occurs because the dog's heart fails.

Absorption of the toxin into the dog's system is rapid, and researchers report that Florida's version of the poisonous toad appears to produce more potent toxin than do *Bufo marinus* found in other areas such as Hawaii or Texas.

If a dog owner suspects a dog has encountered a poisonous toad, the first step is to promptly wash the dog's mouth out thoroughly with water. Some veterinarians suggest that the dog should be induced to vomit, while others advise hustling the dog to a veterinarian's office as fast as possible after rinsing the dog's mouth.

INSECTS AND ARACHNIDS

During Florida summers, the state seems alive with insects of every assortment. Some of them treat dogs the same way they treat humans—they bite or sting.

Bees, Wasps, and Yellow Jackets

These insects rarely cause serious problems if they sting a dog unless an allergic reaction occurs or if the dog receives numerous stings. Sting sites may become swollen and painful, but ice often provides temporary relief. In the case of bee stings, the owner should

The country dog that tangles with a skunk can be washed in tomato juice and rubbed dry with corn meal. Only time will completely diminish the odor.

The American Kennel Club reports that as of 1988 the most popular
10 dog breeds, in order, were:
1. Cocker spaniel
2. Labrador retriever
3. Poodle
4. Golden retriever
5. German shepherd
6. Chow Chow
7. Rottweiler
8. Beagle
9. Dachshund
10. Miniature schnauzer

remove the stinger, which the bee usually leaves in the dog's skin.

Owners should watch for an allergic reaction to stings that could
send the dog into shock. Initial signs of shock are a whitening of the
gums and rapid breathing and heart rates.

Spiders and Scorpions

Florida has three biting or stinging arachnids that can harm dogs:

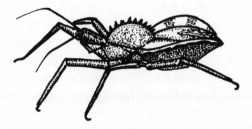

The so-called wheel bug is a grayish-brown insect that blends in with plant matter. Its
name derives from a curved series of "cogs" on its back that resemble a wheel. This
insect is a little over one inch long and feeds primarily on other insects, including
hornworms, Japanese beetles, and caterpillars. It can stab people or animals that
handle it, and a few Florida veterinarians report treating dogs that have encountered
these bugs.

the brown recluse spider, the black widow spider, and the scorpion.

The brown recluse, also called a violin spider, is a dull grayish-brown color. It appears to be (including legs) about the size of a fifty-cent piece. An identifying characteristic found on this spider's back is a fiddle or violin-shaped marking. The "base" of the violin is on the spider's abdomen with the "neck" of the violin on the creature's cephalothorax (head-neck region). Recluse spiders in Florida usually are found outside in debris, or indoors behind furniture or under clutter such as piles of clothing.

Several widow spiders are found in the state. Most people recognize the southern black widow with its glossy "black patent" topside and its vivid orange hourglass on the underside of the abdomen. In Florida, the black widow is primarily the southern variety; its northern cousin is found only in the Panhandle region of the state west of Tallahassee.

Other black widow species in Florida include the red widow and brown widow spiders. These differ in the overall body color and markings. The red widow has no hourglass but may have two red spots on the abdomen. The brown widow does have the familiar hourglass identifier and may have a highly variable abdominal pattern of black, white, red, and yellow markings.

Of biting widows, only the southern black widow is of particular concern—and she is seldom found in homes. Her habitat preference is in discarded building materials, water meter boxes, and under park benches and seawall ledges.

Florida's scorpions are about two inches long, brown, and generally found in woodpiles and under ground litter. Their sting is rarely fatal unless it occurs on the dog's head. All of the above-mentioned creatures have the ability to inflict painful bites or stings. And they produce venom. The brown recluse produces a nerve-damaging toxin that can damage the tissues surrounding the wound. The southern black widow's venom spreads very rapidly and may affect muscles, causing tremors and cramping. The scorpion's venom may cause a painful open sore that is slow to heal.

Initial symptoms of bites from these spiders or scorpions may include shivering and vomiting. The dog should receive prompt veterinary attention.

HAZARDS ON THE BEACH

Jellyfish

Every once in a while, a dog at the beach will encounter the stinging jellyfish. Of these, the blue-colored Portuguese man-of-war is the most treacherous. Man-of-wars tend to appear by hundreds some years, favoring Florida's Atlantic coast.

Humans who have encountered the stinging tentacles of the man-of-war report a nearly unbearable stinging sensation. What's more, they pack a double whammy: the bladder that keeps them afloat in the water contains carbon monoxide that will burn the eyes, while the suspended, ribbonlike tentacles that can trail the gas bladder by forty feet contain beads of a nerve poison that is literally drilled into its victim.

Although the man-of-war sounds like something straight from a Hollywood horror movie, it rarely causes death unless the dog (or its owner) develops an allergy, which shows up usually on the second encounter with one of these water sting nettles.

Other jellyfish to be found in Florida waters include the moon jelly, which is clearish-white colored, and the lion's mane, which has a pink hue. Of the two, it is the moon jelly that will render the most painful sting, although it is rarely fatal.

Few dog–jellyfish encounters occur in the water. Most often, dogs are stung when they sniff around a jellyfish that has washed ashore. Even a "washed-up" man-of-war can cause the hapless canine some painful moments. For this reason, owners should always have either physical or voice command over their dogs while walking along the state's beaches.

Fish Hooks

A number of Florida dogs find themselves "hooked" each year by the barbed ends of fishing lines. This occurs when the dog is swimming near popular fishing areas or by the dog just being in the wrong place when a fishing line is cast. Some dogs enjoy playing with a just-landed fish or eating fish bait, and thus end up getting the hook in their foot or mouth. In severe instances, where the dog actually swallows a fish hook, major surgery to remove the hook from the tongue, throat, esophagus, or stomach may be the only expensive (and risky) recourse.

Prevention is the measure of choice. Keep dogs away from casting anglers, and always cast the line safely away from a four-footed fishing buddy. Never reward Sport with tidbits of fish bait—it's a perilous acquired taste.

POISONOUS PLANTS

Dogs are technically classified as carnivores, that is, meat eaters. Any dog owner can attest, however, that canine palates are wide-ranging, and dogs can be seen chomping insects or even plants.

Fortunately, dogs rarely encounter Florida's poisonous plants. This may be because the nearly infallible canine nose knows best, or because sheer luck prevails. Following is a brief description of Florida's poisonous plants that can affect dogs:

Bagpod This tall (six to twelve feet) annual weed is found nearly all over Florida in old fields and around lakes and savannahs. The plant's stems are fern-looking with ten to twenty-six pairs of leaflets spaced along four- to ten-inch stems. Its poison causes intense inflammation of the digestive tract.

Castor Bean In south Florida the castor bean is a treelike plant, but in other areas it is considered an annual herb. It can grow ten feet tall on its strong stem. Leaves are often immense, up to thirty inches across, and star-shaped with five to nine or more lobes. Flowers emerge from the stem ends in clusters and may be greenish-white to rust-colored. Fruits are spiny, oval-shaped, and either green or red. This is the plant from which castor oil is derived, and it is poisonous if enough of any part of the plant is eaten.

Cocklebur This weedy plant stands one to four feet tall. Its triangle-shaped leaf blades are two to ten inches long, arranged alternately on a stout stalk that may be dotted with dull red color. Its green flowers are barely noticeable compared with the plant's main feature: one-inch-long fruit pods. These oblong pods are either green or brown and covered with hooked stickers. The tip of the fruit bears two prominent spines. Poisoning occurs usually in spring on drained wetlands when plants are in their seedling stage. The plants also thrive in old fields.

Croatalaria   Rife along Florida's roadside, this plant is sometimes purposely planted as a cover crop. It is partial to sandy areas and stands between three and six feet tall, with an erect stem bearing several branches on which leaves of four to seven inches are found. Pea-shaped yellow flowers grow in the upper portions of the stem. This plant produces an alkaloid poisoning that lowers an animal's blood pressure and heart rate.

Dogbane (Bitter Root)   This elegant plant grows five to six feet high. The leaves are oval, two or three inches long. Flowers are bell-shaped and pink. Dogbane is usually found in the dry, sandy regions bordering woods. All parts of this plant exude a milky juice that contains potentially toxic resins and sugar derivatives.

Jimsonweed   A purplish main stem three to five feet tall supports this annual weed. Its leaves are light green, three to eight inches long, and have irregular points forming the shape. Flowers can be either white or pale blue-purple and vaguely resemble morning-glories. Toxins of this plant include atropine and alkaloids, which can cause partial blindness and respiratory failure. Jimsonweed is part of the nightshade family.

Milkweed   Found in Florida's sandy areas, this perennial plant grows one to three feet high. Numerous reddish stems arise from a single white root. Leaves are elongated, hairy, and dark green. Flowers are bright orange, growing in clusters. Known as pleurisy root by old-timers, milkweed forms elongated seed pods that terminate in silky hairs. All parts of the plant can be toxic, producing bloating and loss of bodily control.

Nightshade   Growing year-round in south Florida, nightshade has narrow leaves one to four inches long on short stalks. Flowers are white with a yellow center, star-shaped, and grow in clusters. Blackish-purple berries are produced by the plant. The leaves and berries contain a paralytic poison that does not respond well to medical treatment. These plants are found nearly everywhere in the state except adjacent to salt water.

Oleander   One of the state's most popular landscape plants, oleander can poison humans and animals. It has a large trunk that can grow up to twenty-five feet high and support treelike branches. Leaves on the branches are narrow, three to ten inches long. Its five-petaled flower clusters are white, pink, yellow, rose, or red. Milky toxins exude from this plant.

Rattlebox This shrub can reach a height of ten feet. Its leaves are four to eight inches long and lined with six to twenty pairs of leaflets. The flowers resemble those of the sweet pea and are showy in orangish-red. This attractive plant has been used as an ornamental, especially in north Florida. It can be found around houses and in moist areas near waterways. The most dangerous part of this plant is the seed, which inflames the digestive tract.

Sorghum These grasses can grow to fifteen feet in height, although they are rarely more than eight feet tall. Long, narrow leaves erupt from stem joints. Flowers are clusters found at the end of stems in colors of white, pink, yellow, brown, or reddish-brown. Sorghum is a common feed crop planted in north Florida, which would suggest that it is not toxic. In fact, only under special conditions do the plant's enzymes release a most potent poison, hydrocyanic acid (cyanide). Toxic-producing conditions occur when the plant is enhanced with nitrogen-based fertilizers and when drought conditions stunt the sorghum plants. Death occurs almost instantly to a dog that opts to chew on sorghum that is in the toxic state.

Water Hemlock Found in moist or swampy areas of the state, this shrub resembles parsnip. It is a pleasant-looking plant that ranges from three to six feet in height. Leaves are sharply pointed and toothed with obvious veins. Flowers are small, umbrella-shaped clusters of white that bear a baby's-breath fragility. Water hemlock is one of the most toxic plants on the continent, and just a small amount can cause a painful, convulsive death.

Yellow Jessamine Also called Carolina jessamine, this climbing, yellow vine is not as common in south Florida as it is in the central or northern regions. The plant is a riot of stems and tendrils bearing elongated leaves measuring nearly three inches. The sweet-scented, tubular yellow flowers tend to cluster to form masses of color. This plant contains a toxin that can depress or even paralyze motor nerve endings. If consumed by animal or human it can affect vision and produce respiratory problems.

As previously mentioned, most Florida dogs seem to sense which plants are dangerous. Few cases of plant poisonings are reported.

However, some dogs, let to run and desperately hungry, may attempt to eat a poisonous plant. Dogs that dig through garbage for scraps may also encounter poisonous yard clippings that include oleander.

CHEMICAL POISONING

Far more apt than plants to poison Florida dogs are dangerous chemicals used by gardeners and farmers or those toxins encountered in a polluted water source. A little-known source of poisoning can be as close as the manicured local park. Some owners have noticed their dogs becoming ill after spending time in certain parks; the problem often can be traced to weed-killing herbicides.

One of the most common poisons affecting dogs is lead, probably because bored or hungry dogs will occasionally find old linoleum, chunks of plaster, and even peeling paint to chew. Younger animals are more affected by lead than older dogs. Initial symptoms of lead poisoning are listlessness or excitability and convulsive seizures. Veterinary treatment is often successful if exposure to the lead source has not been long term.

Another chemical that dogs may encounter is strychnine. This is often the poison of choice for malicious people who want to get rid of a neighbor's pet. It is found in rat poison, and farm dogs can be poisoned directly by eating the bait or by eating a rat that has been poisoned. Symptoms of strychnine poisoning don't usually appear for about an hour and vary with the amount of strychnine consumed. Initial signs include nervousness, muscle stiffness, and a rabid-doglike response to bright light or loud noise. The dog may grow rigid and stand like a sawhorse. Violent spasms may begin and breathing may become difficult, even ceasing for seconds at a time. If left unattended, the dog eventually dies of exhaustion in less than two hours.

Metaldehyde and N-methyl carbamates used with bran in some snail baits are another common poison affecting dogs. The symptoms closely resemble those of strychnine poisoning. Fortunately, fewer manufacturers are using the formulas that dogs found so tasty, so the number of carbamate poisonings is declining.

A fairly common dog poison is found in most Florida garages—ethylene glycol, more commonly called antifreeze. Dogs like its sweet taste, and male dogs tend to be more commonly affected than females.

As with other poisons, antifreeze induces vomiting, nausea, depression, and increased thirst. In addition, the dog may have trouble standing. In more severe cases, the dog will convulse and the heart will beat irregularly.

Veterinarians report that many dog owners do not notice the initial poisoning symptoms of antifreeze. It is not until twenty-four to seventy-two hours later, when the dog's ailments have become more severe, that an owner decides something is wrong and scoots off to the veterinary clinic. This poisoning can be successfully treated if begun before vital organs such as the kidney and heart become involved.

Sweet taste attracts dogs to another poisoning that most dog owners would never guess: chocolate poisoning. Researchers say that animal poison control centers report a high incidence of chocolate toxicosis, and in some cases the dogs have died. The culprit is a compound called theobromine, found naturally in chocolate and tea. Closely related, but not causing any notable number of canine deaths, is caffeine poisoning. Both chocolate and caffeine cause restlessness, irregular heartbeat, muscle tremors, and seizures.

As soon as an owner recognizes the symptoms of chocolate or caffeine poisoning, the dog should be taken to the veterinarian. The best treatment is afforded within two hours after the onset of symptoms. There is no specific antidote, so veterinarians strive to get the dog's stomach emptied and to stabilize the condition.

A rarer dog poison is aflatoxins, a toxic mold found on peanuts, rice, corn, and other cereals. Signs of this poison are at first subtle, a barely noticeable loss of a dog's healthy condition. By the time an owner recognizes a severe decline in the dog's health, it is usually too late.

66 There's a hope for every woe, and a balm for every pain.
—Robert Gilfillan 99

CHAPTER **9**

Pooch Patching

A knowledgeable dog owner is one who inevitably spends less time visiting—and paying—veterinarians. That owner also saves its dog a lot of needless suffering.

Nevertheless, dogs, especially puppies, are curious and playful and can get into instant trouble. The advice in this chapter is intended to offer only temporary assistance to owners whose dogs have been injured or involved in some kind of accident. An injured animal should be seen as soon as possible by a veterinarian, particularly if the pet shows signs of going into shock.

DROWNING

Florida dogs, like their owners, enjoy a life that often includes boat rides or trips to fishing or swimming holes. Dogs are adequate paddling swimmers, but if they must swim long distances or if the water is rough, they can drown from exhaustion.

The obvious first step in rescuing an apparently drowned dog is to fish it from the water. Once it is out of the water, hold the dog up by its hind legs, head down, and drain the water from its mouth. If the dog is a large breed and difficult to hold upside-down, find a locale where the dog can be laid with hindquarters higher than its head so the water can drain out.

Check the animal's respiration and heartbeat. If the dog has no heartbeat, the heart can be artificially stimulated similar to the method used on humans. A dog's heart is situated in generally the same spot as a human's. Press gently about once per second in the heart region.

If the dog's heart is beating but the animal is not breathing, blow gently into the dog's nostrils while holding its mouth shut. The proper speed is about once every three seconds. Resuscitation is best done with the dog lying flat on its back or on its side. Heart stimulation should be alternated with artificial respiration and continued until the dog revives or until it is decided that the dog cannot be helped.

A revived dog may still suffer from shock. Its gums may be pale and a rapid heartbeat (more than 150 beats per minute) may begin. If that is the case, wrap the dog in warm towels or blankets and get the animal to a veterinarian as quickly as possible.

ELECTRICAL SHOCK

Puppies or bored adult dogs may include electrical cords among their chew toys. If the dog contacts a live wire, the dog may try vainly to free itself of the cord but will be unable to because it is frozen to the current surge. The dog may even be knocked unconscious

> **Shock is the number one killer of dogs that have been involved in accidents.**

if the cord insulation was bitten through. Never touch a dog if the electrical cord is still in the animal's mouth. First unplug the cord, then tend the animal.

Check the animal's breathing. If it is breathing, examine the mouth for electrical burns and wash the mouth out with water or with a solution of equal parts of water with 3 percent hydrogen peroxide.

If the animal is not breathing, check for a heartbeat. If a beat is heard or felt, place the dog on its side and begin artificial respiration (see the previous section on drowning). Check periodically to see if the dog has begun breathing. If not, continue artificial respiration. If there is no heartbeat, initiate cardiopulmonary resuscitation (again, see the previous section). Continue until the dog is revived.

Shock is the next danger that can kill the revived dog. As mentioned earlier, if the animal's gums grow pale and a rapid heartbeat is noted, the dog should be gathered up and taken to a veterinarian. But before racing off to the doctor, put a wrapped hot water bottle against the dog's stomach area and swaddle the animal in a blanket or towel.

If a dog fully recovers from the immediate crisis, there may be problems later as tissues affected by the electrical trauma die off. The veterinarian is the best source of help.

FISH HOOK REMOVAL

The first rule in dealing with fish hooks is to know when and when not to remove them. If the hook is embedded in the dog's tongue or the roof of the mouth, do not attempt to remove it yourself. Seek medical help instead.

A second rule is to know whether restraining the animal is necessary. Many a frightened, injured dog will bite at the nearest object, even its owner. It may be a good idea to wrap a piece of cloth securely around the dog's muzzle to keep it from biting in panic.

If the fish hook is lodged in the dog's skin, or in the outer area of the mouth, use a pair of pliers to ease the hook toward whatever direction makes the barbs clear the skin. Lop off the barbs with a wire or hook cutter and slip the hook out of the skin in the direction it entered. Next, thoroughly clean the wound with hydrogen peroxide. If the wound bleeds, press some sterile gauze on it until it stops.

HEAT STROKE

Anytime a dog is kept where it cannot keep its body temperature at proper coolness, it will suffer heat stroke (hyperthermia). In Florida, closed-up cars are the most frequent offenders—and leaving a dog in that situation is as cruel as putting it in an oven.

Signs of heat stroke are collapse and rapid or deep breathing. The dog may appear to be staring out into space, it may be vomiting or suffering diarrhea, and the mouth is a vivid red color.

If an overheated dog is discovered, rapid action is required. Once a dog has reached the point of obvious debilitation, it takes only several more minutes before it will suffer brain damage and die. Therefore, cool the dog's body as fast as possible. The best option is to immerse the dog in a tub of cold water; the second best treatment is to run cold water over it from a hose. Once the dog's whole body has been doused, concentrate on the pulse points such as around the tail, the legs, and stomach. This should be continued for a half-hour. Ice packs may be used around the dog's head. Once the dog has revived, take it to a veterinarian for a thorough checkup.

POISONING

Occasionally a vicious soul decides to get rid of perceived canine pests with poison. Then there are curious dogs who accidentally poison themselves. Once poisoning, by whatever means, is discovered, quick action is vital.

Carbon monoxide poisoning: Occurs occasionally, usually when a dog is transported in the trunk of a car, an inhumane practice. Exhaust fumes leak into the trunk and overcome the dog. Cardio-pulmonary resuscitation and administering oxygen are necessary as soon as possible, or the dog could die from insufficient oxygen to the brain. Symptoms are deep red gums, heavy breathing, weakness, and convulsions.

Flea collar poisoning: Occurs rarely, but occasionally accounts for unexplained illness in dogs. It generally occurs when a flea dip or shampoo containing one type of insecticide is used in conjunction with a collar containing another type of insecticide. If a dog wears a collar, it is a good idea to check with a veterinarian about the best type of dip or shampoo to use. Similarly, if a flea-inhibiting medication is being given, check with the doctor to see if use of the flea collar offers any chemical conflict.

Garbage poisoning: Dogs are carrion eaters from 10,000 years back. Occasionally, however, they overdo it and the vomiting mechanism fails to clear the plumbing. Bacteria that bakes in garbage under the Florida sun can overwhelm the dog, which exhibits the usual signs of poisoning: abdominal pain, diarrhea, vomiting, and occasionally paralysis. In mild instances, an oral dose of Epsom salts, one teaspoon to a small quantity of water, can help the dog clear the offending toxins from the gastrointestinal tract. If these measures fail to perk up the dog, take it to the veterinarian along with a sample of the vomit material.

Herbicide poisoning (wood preservatives, weed killers): May be encountered along roadways where utility companies spray to keep vines away from power or telephone lines, or in city parks that use sprays to keep invading weeds in check. Generally, doses that are publicly used would cause only mild illness, but owners should be aware of these toxins in case the dog is suffering an ailment for which no cause can be found. Symptoms include loss of appetite, restlessness, and muscle tremors. Extreme illness from herbicide exposure also includes convulsions. It is unlikely that an owner would know the specific herbicide involved, so it is best to take the dog to the veterinarian.

Pesticide poisoning (snail or roach baits, insect sprays): Usually consumed by a curious or hungry dog or when a dog licks the material from its paws or fur. Signs are trembling, vomiting, weakness, abdominal pain, frothing at the mouth, and convulsions. If the dog has not vomited, induce with one teaspoon per ten pounds of body weight of 3 percent hydrogen peroxide, which should be given once every ten minutes. Keep the dog quiet and warm and transport it to a veterinarian as quickly as possible.

Petroleum poisoning (paint or cleaning solvents, kerosene): The

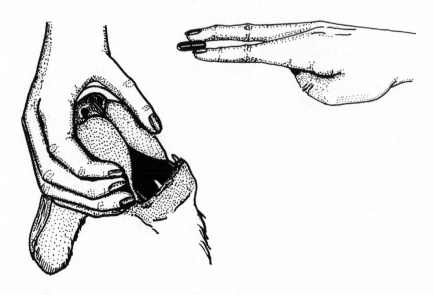

To "pill" a dog, press gently on its muzzle to prompt it to open its mouth. Place the pill in the dog's mouth as far back on the tongue as possible, close the dog's mouth, and gently hold it closed while stroking the throat to encourage swallowing. By holding the pill as illustrated (right), it is possible to place the pill deep into the dog's mouth.

dog's gums will grow pale; its heartbeat and breathing will grow more rapid. Lips or other skin on the animal's body may be blistered. The first step is to get the chemical out of the dog's mouth. Wash out the mouth, holding the animal's head down to discourage swallowing and so the animal does not choke on the water. Do not give the dog anything to make it vomit; that would further damage the mouth and esophagus tissues as the material re-enters the mouth from the stomach. Next, call either a veterinarian's office or a poison control center to learn if there is an antidote. If the dog is convulsing, wrap it in a blanket and take it to a veterinarian.

Poisonous plant poisoning: Relatively rare, but signs of weakness, abdominal pain, frothing at the mouth, and lack of coordination indicate the dog may have eaten a poisonous plant. Induce vomiting with a teaspoon of 3 percent hydrogen peroxide given every ten minutes until vomiting occurs. This can be followed by a teaspoonful of Epsom salts and water, which empties the intestine. This treatment usually improves the dog's condition, but if breathing difficulties or convulsions begin, take the dog to a veterinarian.

Rodenticide poisoning: Consumed by the dog either firsthand, from eating mouse or rat bait, or by eating a dead rodent. Signs of poisoning may differ because there are many types of rodenticides on the market. Many of the most common of these poisons prevent blood from clotting. As a result, a dog who has eaten any of these poisons may suffer internal bleeding. Owners who suspect their dog has consumed rodent poison should immediately consult a veterinarian. If possible, give the veterinarian the poison's brand name.

POISONOUS SNAKE AND INSECT BITES

Florida's snakes and spiders can inflict painful and even lethal bites. Fortunately, few dogs are bitten by such creatures, and those who are rarely die.

Dogs that have been bitten by a poisonous snake exhibit such symptoms as weakness, nausea, paralysis, impaired vision, and swelling. A common side effect of snakebites is the dying off of tissues surrounding the wound. This may go on for days.

Veterinarians recommend placing ice around the bite site to slow the dispersal of venom in the dog's system. Above all, quickly move the dog to a source of antivenin. It's helpful to know the type of snake that bit the dog so the proper antivenin can be used.

Some books advise first-aid procedures such as cutting and orally sucking the venom from the wound. This can be dangerous for at least three reasons. First, a cut to a site near an artery could cause the dog to bleed to death before reaching the veterinarian's office. Second, if there is a raw spot on the owner's lips or in the mouth, the venom could enter the owner's bloodstream. Third, the administration

The normal, healthy dog has the following vital signs:
Temperature: 100–102 degrees Fahrenheit
Pulse Rate: 100–130 beats per minute
Respiration: 22 breaths per minute

of first aid by an untrained person will delay moving the dog to the chief source of help, antivenin.

Similarly, the bites of some spiders (such as the black widow or the brown recluse) as well as a sting from a scorpion can cause poisoning. First-aid methods for shock should be used and the dog should be taken to the veterinarian immediately.

SHOCK

Not to be confused with electrical shock, this type of shock refers to the signs that the dog's body is beginning to weaken and the dog is nearing death due to the failure of blood flowing to body tissues.

At the onset, shock induces the heart to accelerate and the blood vessels constrict, so the dog's pulse rate races while its gums appear pale. If treatment is delayed, shock reaction shifts into another gear—the dog's poor circulation deprives the heart of blood, the animal weakens, outer blood vessels begin to dilate (which further weakens the heart), and the body's acidity begins to change. At some point, depending on the animal's health and age and the seriousness of the injury, death occurs.

The goal when treating an animal suffering from shock is to get it to the veterinarian quickly so drugs, blood, electrolytes, and other lifesaving measures can be administered. On the way, try keeping the dog's hindquarters propped higher than its head to keep blood circulating to the brain. Keep the dog warm with a hot water bottle and blankets.

Animals recovering from shock may have to be left at the veterinarian's clinic for observation because relapses can occur.

STINGS

Insect stings occasionally bother Florida dogs. Most bites result in nothing more than a swollen area, but dogs that receive a number of bites from bees, wasps, or yellow jackets, or dogs that are allergic to such bites, may develop a reaction termed anaphylactic shock.

Symptoms of this problem include diarrhea, vomiting, and increased salivation. Many veterinarians recommend giving the dog a human cold capsule that contains antihistimines, while others say such drugs have little effect. Again, getting the dog to a veterinarian is important,

Recommended Canine Medicine Chest

Medications

Boric acid eye wash	Hydrogen peroxide (3%)
Antiseptic powder	Petroleum jelly
Antibacterial ointment	Mild laxative (human)
Mild antidiarrhea medicine	Blood-clotting powder

Equipment

Adhesive tape	Gauze
Sterile gauze pads	Safety pins
Muslin strips (3 feet long)	Dose syringes or eyedroppers
Ice bags or packs	Blanket and towels
Tweezers	4 to 5 feet of nylon rope
Cotton swabs	Scissors (stitch removing)
Thermometer (rectal)	Paint-mixing stick splints

Keep the above medications and equipment packed in a box so that whatever is needed can be grabbed in an emergency.

and the dog may be aided in travel by raising the hindquarters higher than the head and by keeping the animal warm.

In the event the dog does not have a reaction to the bite but is in obvious pain, diluted ammonia may ease the stinging sensation.

A dog may exhibit reaction to jellyfish stings, especially if a man-of-war has been encountered. The painful sting may be alleviated with diluted ammonia. If the dog exhibits a severe reaction, the animal should be transported to the veterinarian's office for treatment of anaphylactic shock.

RESTRAINING AN INJURED DOG

Man's best friend can turn into a frenzied stranger when in pain or terribly frightened. If the dog seems vicious, it is wise to restrain the animal.

Carefully observe the dog as you approach it. If it is growling or behaving threateningly, slip a strip of cloth, a belt, or anything else that is handy around the dog's neck. The objective is to subdue the dog's head so that a strip of cloth or rope can be tied around the muzzle to keep the mouth closed and unable to bite.

If the dog is a Pekingese or some other type of snub-nosed dog, muzzling will not work, so toss a blanket or towel completely over the dog and wrap it up so it can be carried.

Caution should be used when muzzling a dog because it cannot breathe as well with its mouth clamped shut. And if the dog is vomiting, it could choke to death. In cases where the dog is straining to breathe or is vomiting, bundle it up in a blanket or towel and get to a veterinarian.

If the dog has been hit by a car or is believed to have broken bones, it should be immobilized by placing it on a board or other flat surface and restrained by tying a blanket around it. Do not tie the dog to the flat surface near its neck—confine the restraints to the torso area.

Unaltered male dogs can be very territorial. The result can be dogfights, causing injuries to people who try to separate the sparring animals. Human interference is often unnecessary for two reasons: most dogs sense that a graceful exit is the better part of valor so they seldom fight to the death, and dogfights generally sound worse than they are. Attempts to break up a fight usually work best if the more aggressive dog can be distracted long enough to allow the weaker dog to escape. A dousing with a garden hose may accomplish this. In extremely serious situations, where a larger (possibly rabid) dog has cornered a smaller one, a phone call to either the dog control officials or the police may be in order.

Once the dust settles, a dog that has been seriously injured should be taken to the veterinarian to protect it against bite infections and as a precaution against rabies. Properly handling the injured dog and guarding it against going into shock are the best first-aid measures.

VOMITING

Vomiting is nature's way of keeping the dog healthy by ridding it of offensive materials it may have eaten. Dogs that run loose may frequently vomit because they dine at the curbside cafeteria and consume some fairly unspeakable items, but continued vomiting may indicate more than an upset stomach. For instance, kidney, liver, and pancreas problems may prompt vomiting, as can viral infections. If vomiting continues for hours and contains no blood, the owner should place Fido in an easily cleaned locale such as a utility room or bathroom and keep food and water away for twelve hours. A stomach-coating human medication can be used to help settle the animal's digestive tract.

Following the twelve-hour fast, the dog may have a little water. If the vomiting seems to have abated, try small amounts of soft, bland food such as water-soaked bread, cottage cheese, or cooked rice. Regular feeding can be slowly resumed over several days.

Make sure the vomiting is not caused by a chunk of bone or other obstruction that has lodged in the dog's throat. If there is any blood present, make sure a veterinarian sees the dog pronto. Do not ignore

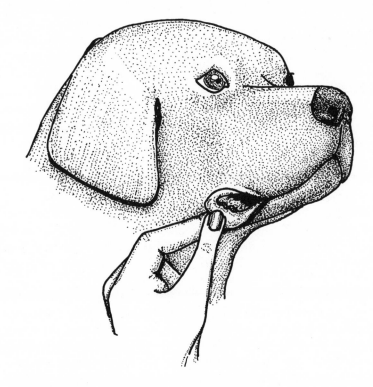

Dogs can be given liquid medicine easily. Gently pull out a fold of the corner of the mouth and squirt medication in with a syringe or dropper.

chronic vomiting for more than twenty-four hours because the dog can suffer severe electrolyte loss and life-threatening dehydration.

It cannot be emphasized enough that injured or ill dogs should be seen by a qualified veterinarian. Many ailments and injuries resemble each other and can be misdiagnosed by the dog owner. For example, a dog that is frothing at the mouth may be suffering from poisoning or from heat stroke. Similarly, a convulsing dog may be suffering an injury, may be having an epileptic seizure, may be suffering heat stroke, or may have a bone caught in its throat.

In any emergency, the best advice to an owner is to stay calm, evaluate the situation, stabilize the dog if possible, and get prompt medical attention for the stricken animal.

I'm a lean dog, a keen
dog, a wild dog, and lone;
I'm a rough dog, a tough
dog, hunting on my own;
I'm a bad dog, a mad dog,
teasing silly sheep;
I love to sit and bay the
moon, to keep fat souls
from sleep.
　　　　—Irene McLeod

CHAPTER

10

Of Buffets and Baths

Nutritional requirements for Florida dogs are the same as for dogs anywhere. What most dog owners may notice, however, is that the heat and humidity may decrease the dog's activity, and so less food for more mature dogs may be in order.

PUPPY NUTRITION

Proper nutrition is most important for growing puppies. Up to about three or four weeks of age, puppies stick pretty much to mother's milk. Soft, solid food may interest the youngster, and at about age six to eight weeks the puppy will wean itself from mom to meat.

Many breeders will feed puppies at will, giving the young dog about as much to eat as it wants. Dry food should be moistened with water for the first six months. After that age, as the puppy matures to about fifteen to eighteen months, the dog can be fed twice a day.

The quantity fed depends on the pup's breed and body size. Obviously, a smaller dog eats less than a large dog. A six-month-old, medium-sized puppy that weighs around 20 pounds should get 1,050 calories a day, about three cups of nutritionally complete puppy chow.

ADULT DOG NUTRITION

Once the puppy is mature (at ten months for small breeds to fifteen or eighteen months for the larger breeds), it is ready for adult dog diets.

The primary difference between puppy and adult dog diet is calories. Puppies are growing and more active, so they require about twice the adult dog's intake of calories. A balanced adult dog formula of canned, moist, or dry food can be fed twice a day, but it's a good idea to feed at the same time each day.

WHAT'S COOKING?

For many dogs, what the owner eats is what Rover gets, too. But breeders and veterinarians agree that table scraps can impair the balance of a dog's diet and can cause a dog to become a downright picky eater. Scraps can be added to balanced foods but should be less than 15 percent of the dog's diet. If a dog is nursing puppies, she should receive additional food.

Commercial Dog Food

Prepared or commercial dog food comes in a variety of styles:

Dry food takes the form of pellets, flakes, or chunks and usually provides about 80 percent of a dog's needed nutrition. And, because dry foods are just that—dry—they provide more nutrition pound for pound than any other type of food. They are also convenient to store. In Florida, it is a good idea not to buy in such large quantities that supplies remain around (unless sealed in their original bags) more than several weeks. Otherwise, mold, mildew, and bugs can invade.

Moist foods are a dry food that contain from 25 to 40 percent moisture, which can leave the food soon after the package is opened. Because they contain moisture, they often also contain spoilage retardants to fight bacteria and fungi. There are reports that some moist food formulas can cause a dog's urine to become acidic. Don't be fooled by the hamburgerlike processing of moist foods; although enjoyed by many dogs and convenient to use, such foods consist primarily of meat and bone meal with soybean meal and sugar, with added vitamins and minerals.

Canned foods are probably the least convenient form of dog food and must be refrigerated after opening. They generally contain as much as nearly 80 percent water. Few are 100 percent pure meat. Those that are labeled "beef" or "liver" contain about 95 percent of those primary ingredients. The remainder is added vitamins and minerals. A label that indicates the can is a "gourmet beef buffet" or a "luscious liver dinner" or some other generic dining term means that it contains only about 25 percent of the principal ingredient. Canned food labeled "beef flavored" or "liver flavored" means that the mystery meat is enhanced with those flavors, although the beef in "beef flavored" may be discerned only by the most astute canine nose.

No matter what choice of feeding the owner elects, the dog should have free access to clean water. Dry food in particular may prompt the dog to drink a large quantity of water, and if denied, the dog could become dehydrated.

Also, the dog or puppy's food dish should be routinely cleaned. Dry food, as mentioned, can develop mold and mildew; wet food can grow rancid. Perhaps a more repellent thought: Florida's behemoth cockroaches simply adore dog food leftovers.

Treats

Name a shape and there is probably a doggie treat to fit it. Little bones, fish, cheeses, miniature dogs, cats, even human shapes—all are aimed at appealing not to dogs, but to dog owners. Fortunately (and despite the anthropomorphism), most dog treats are nutritionally well balanced and serve to reward the dog as well as to provide

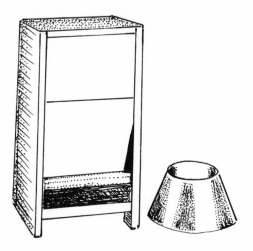

Two feeding options are the automatic feeding bin (left), which permits the dog to eat at will, and the "spaniel bowl" (right), designed to keep long-eared breeds from dipping their ear tips in the food or water.

another form of nourishment. A benefit to teeth is provided by some treats that must be chewed.

Supplements

Unless recommended by a veterinarian to treat a specific ailment, most dogs do not need vitamin or mineral supplements as long as they are fed a high-quality balanced diet. Do not feed dogs any supplements designed for humans because a canine's needs differ from those of people. For example, few dogs benefit from vitamin C. Indeed, most dogs rarely suffer from vitamin or mineral deficiencies unless they are fed virtually nothing but table scraps that have lost vitamins and minerals during cooking.

Bones to Pick

Some dogs will kill for milk. But the sugar (lactose) in milk is difficult for some dogs to digest. The lactose may ferment in the intestinal tract and cause the dog problems with gas and diarrhea.

Similarly, save the chicken, fish, sparerib, and pork chop bones for the garbage disposal or the compost pile. Dogs do not digest these bones well. Worse, the bones can splinter and puncture the dog's mouth, stomach, or intestinal wall. The result is at the very least an excruciatingly painful experience for your pet. The effect on your wallet after the vet bill arrives will not feel so good either.

Hearty beef bones are best—the versions that are large enough that the dog cannot swallow any portion whole. There was a fond time when butchers would just hand such bony leftovers to a customer, but now they cost money. Still, they help keep the dog's teeth clean and provide hours of amusement for the stay-at-home dog.

FIDO FATTIES

An overweight dog is an unhealthy dog. And, say some veterinary surveys, about 40 percent of the nation's canines are overweight. Some veterinarians are downright blunt about pointing out dog paunch. A few veterinarians will venture as far as "Well, well, Rover's certainly grown since he was last here," and hope the owner takes a hint. A few others, though, have seen enough "insulted" clients huff right out the door, their pets waddling behind, to broach the subject of obesity.

One University of Florida veterinarian who specializes in dog obesity says knowing when Rover's rotund figure should be curbed is easy: "Run your hands gently along the dog's sides. If you cannot feel the ribs, then the dog's too heavy." Grossly obese dogs are those who resemble barrels on legs. "Some breeds such as Labradors, cocker spaniels, and beagles tend to put weight on easily," he says. With those breeds, genetics is doing its bit to turn every tidbit into tonnage. The fact is, carrying too much weight around, particularly in Florida's heat and humidity, can shorten a dog's life. To wit, the obesity specialist says that many Florida dog owners are literally "feeding their dogs to death."

Roly-poly puppies, while adorable, also can develop bone problems from carrying too much excess weight. Adult dogs may develop joint troubles, breathing difficulties, digestive problems, and even higher rates of canine cancers.

One obvious answer to getting the fat off is to cut back calories and increase exercise. That is often difficult. Dogs tend to grow sluggish with age and calories need to be cut back without sacrificing nutrition. The same can be said for dogs that are cooped up in apartments all day. Those factors, combined with many dogs' "live to eat" mentality, make calorie cutting a real chore. Some dogs have an uncanny ability to snitch snacks—a chunk of the cat's dinner here, a guest's potato chip there.

The university specialist advises owners to monitor their dog's eating habits more closely. Simply cutting back on the amount a dog is fed may leave the animal unhappily hungry, so the answer may be in the new lines of "lite" dog food increasingly available on the pet shelves of grocery stores. These diet brands generally contain from 15 to 25 percent fewer calories.

A second aid in getting the weight off of chubby canines is to increase the amount of exercise. Most owners also benefit by a longer walk on balmy Florida evenings. Other good exercises include swimming and making a game out of exercising by training the dog to play with a ball or a Frisbie.

GROOMING THE FLORIDA DOG

Florida's climate and the state's abundant supply of insects offer plenty of grooming headaches to dog owners. Many dog owners resort to frequent bathing of their dogs, particularly of the Fidos who live indoors. Indeed, frequent bathing makes a dog more pleasant to live with, but such cleanliness may not be in the best interest of the dog's skin.

Imagine for a moment that the area under the dog's coat can be viewed with magnified vision. The scene would be a tiny ecology of regenerating skin tissues—old cells sloughing off (dandruff) and being replaced by new ones. Microscopic creatures work to keep the skin and hair follicles in top operating balance by aiding in the removal of dead skin and hair. The hair follicles are constantly growing new hairs and shedding out the worn.

In the healthy dog, the skin and hair are kept naturally oiled by normal skin secretions. Frequent baths—one or more a week—can disrupt this normal skin environment. Most soaps will remove too much oil, leaving the skin dry and the coat dull and brittle. Dry-

Bloat is a sometimes fatal intestinal disorder that can affect the best-cared-for dogs, especially large breeds. The exact cause is unkown, but dogs such as setters and Doberman pinschers are among those likely to develop the ailment. The following tips have been found to help prevent bloat:
  —Feed smaller rations two or three times daily.
  —Make sure plenty of water is available to the dog.
  —Use care when changing from one brand of cereal-based food to another.
  —Watch the dog after it eats and look for evidence of abdominal fullness, whining, restlessness, anxiety, and any unsuccessful attempts at vomiting.
  —Delay vigorous exercise until two hours after meals and do not feed the dog for an hour after a strenuous outing.
  —Be especially vigilant while traveling with the dog or after the dog has been boarded.

skinned dogs will scratch just as though they have fleas or a skin ailment.

Daily brushing is best. It keeps skin clean without disrupting the normal function of healthy skin. Another advantage to daily brushing is that it keeps loose, shedded hair to a minimum. Dogs normally shed twice a year, fall and spring, although indoor dogs, especially those in air conditioning, may shed year-round. Longhaired dogs may be groomed with a wire-toothed comb or brush, although care should be taken not to scratch the dog's skin. A natural-bristle brush is sufficient for shorthaired dogs, which can be rubbed down afterward with a clean towel to remove dead hair and skin. Much of the "dog odor" will go into the washing machine with the towel, and the dog's coat will glisten.

That is not to say a dog should not be bathed. For just as humans have distinctive body odors, so do dogs. And that "dogaroma" drives some fastidious owners crazy. However, dog baths should be kept to the minimum number that keeps odors and insects at bay while maintaining the integrity of the dog's skin and coat.

Numerous gentle grooming soaps are available for dogs. They are preferable to human shampoos, which can produce allergic reactions

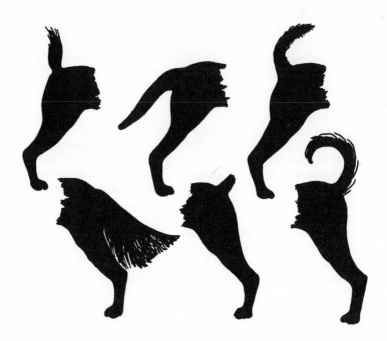

Some canine tail types (clockwise from lower right): ring tail, docked tail, plume tail, gay tail, otter tail, and sickle tail.

due to perfumes or colorings that are added to please people. Similarly, dog shampoos that contain pesticides, alcohol, iodine, or pine tar derivatives should be used as infrequently as possible. Fleas can develop immunity to a preventative product that is used constantly. Other problems are associated with some shampoo additives, too. Alcohol, for example, can dry skin out quickly. And iodine or pine tar products, usually used to clear up particular problems, can be too harsh for healthy-skinned dogs.

Many dog owners dry their dogs with blow dryers. Those that do should keep the heat setting low; if not, the warm air will dry out a dog's coat. The result will be an "itchy" pet whose coat sheds easily and appears dull.

A dog who harbors an unusually offensive odor may need a veterinary inspection more than it needs a bath. Hormone imbalances, allergies, or nutritional deficiencies can spawn pungent odors.

How to Bathe

Begin the bath by dampening around the dog's head to prevent any fleas from seeking refuge inside the dog's ears. Care should be taken to avoid getting soapy water in the dog's eyes or ears. While most dog bathing products do no harm, the dog who makes the connection between burning eyes and baths will soon become less cooperative.

Gently clean the dog's ears but only as deep as can be seen. Swabs or other objects may push wax into the ear canal.

Next, scrub the dog's body. A rubber mitt with a pebbly texture cleans effectively, and most dogs enjoy the massage that comes with a bath. Don't overdo it, though, for keeping the soap on the dog's skin for many minutes will aid in drying it out.

Once the bath is finished, thoroughly dry the dog with towels or a blow dryer set to low and held about twelve inches from the dog.

Grooming the Feet

Owners often find that the bath and drying pretty well exhaust the dog's attention span. Of course, the dog's patience will increase with age, and it soons becomes a handy grooming practice to teach the dog to have its toenails clipped after the bath. This is not only convenient, but the nails are not as brittle after being wetted and they are clean, which makes it easier to see how far down on the nail to trim before hitting the painful (and bloody) arteries known as the quick.

A variety of clippers are available to assist in properly trimming dog toenails. If the quick is accidentally nicked and begins bleeding, use a styptic pencil or a blood-clotting powder available at most pet stores to staunch the flow.

If the dog stays outside or frequently runs in the woods, always check the foot pads for cuts or thorns.

Caring for Teeth

A dog with bad breath can indeed wilt flowers. Check the animal's teeth. Like human teeth, a dog's teeth develop tartar, cavities, and gum problems that result in tooth loss.

Brushing a dog's teeth is possible, and if begun early in the dog's training regimen, it is an effective way to protect the animal's teeth

> Beware of the cute little hair bows placed in the hair of poodles and other dog breeds. If the dog's skin is accidentally bound up in the band, blood circulation can be stopped. If the situation goes unnoticed for long enough, severe damage can result to the blood-starved skin and surgery may be necessary to repair the area.

and prevent bad breath. A child's toothbrush fits nicely into the dog's mouth. Some pet owners use toothpaste and some dogs seem to like the sweet taste, but brushing with baking soda is effective, too.

Neglected teeth may spell a trip to a veterinarian who will clean the dog's choppers with dental instruments.

66Recollect that the Almighty, who gave the dog to be the companion of our pleasures and our toils, hath invested him with a nature noble and incapable of deceit.
*—Sir Walter Scott*99

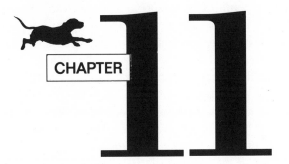

CHAPTER

11

Minding the Manners

T here are many excellent and thorough dog training books as well as many excellent Florida dog trainers to provide useful information about dog handling. But a few major points can help an owner with a new dog if the pet is too young to enroll in a training class.

> A key to training a puppy is repetition, praise for good behavior, and verbal reprimand for bad behavior. Consistency, say trainers, is another must. Always use the same command words and give praise (or if absolutely necessary, punishment) promptly. Young dogs especially do not associate reward or punishment if either is meted out more than a few seconds after the behavior occurs.

HOUSEBREAKING

Usually the first and most critical need of the owner with a new puppy is a few tips on housebreaking. A puppy that must answer nature's call every couple of hours can wreak havoc on carpeting or wood flooring in a mere twenty-four hours. That does not have to happen, but preventing it is up to the owner.

First, an owner needs to know that puppies under twelve weeks old cannot remain continent for much longer than about two hours. For that reason, the owner should choose whether to paper train an indoor dog, or get the pup accustomed to the great outdoors.

When the puppy first comes home, it is essential for outdoor toilet training to take the dog out about once an hour and right after meals. A puppy eight weeks or older is capable of beginning to associate outdoors with voiding. Younger dogs usually are not mentally ready to make such associations, so the outdoor trips are for the protection of the house as well as for the owner's peace of mind. Once the dog is old enough to know what it is going outside to do, the handler should stay there until something is accomplished. It is surprising how quickly most pups begin getting the idea, especially if they are praised when their job is done. They will be further inspired by the aroma of past performances if the handler takes them to the same location each time.

Indoors, stay vigilant. If the puppy starts sniffing around the house, and more than an hour or so has passed since the last elimination, play it safe. Take the pup to a designated "bathroom newspaper." Praise any accomplishments and allow the pup to rejoin the family group after using the "bathroom." At night, place the pup in its sleeping quarters (yes, on newspapers), but arrange it so that it adjoins the newspaper "bathroom." The dog soon will learn where to soil.

Some puppies, if kept constantly only on newspapered areas, never make a clear distinction between the "bathroom newspaper" and any other indoor flooring. To them, every place is eligible for soiling.

All puppies have accidents. When one occurs, scold "No" with the voice, scoop up the pup, and place it in its bathroom area, whether outside or inside. Unfortunately, this only works if the accident is promptly discovered or if the pup is caught in the act. After a few minutes, the dog has forgotten all about soiling, and thus correction is futile. Never overpunish a dog by shoving its nose in the soil or beating it with a newspaper. In fact, making a dog afraid of newspaper could actually inspire the dog to avoid soiling on newspaper.

Many dog owners report success through use of a key command that is used in connection with elimination. For instance, one owner uses the dainty term "tinkle" when her dog is voiding. Using the word while the dog is in the process helps connect the performance with the word. When the dog finishes, it is praised profusely, again using the term. In addition, on every trip outdoors, whether for elimination or not, the friend used the term "out" with the dog. It took about a month, but she succeeded in connecting the two terms "out-tinkle," and the dog realized that going outside was related to nature calls. Now that the dog is grown, all the owner has to do is ask the dog, "Out-tinkle?" If the dog has to eliminate, it responds by going to the door to go outside.

Paper training similarly can be keyed to a certain command word. It should be used every time the puppy is placed on the newspaper. It does not take long, if the owner is consistent, for the pup to make the connection between voiding and the newspaper.

Undoubtedly, positive reinforcement works better than punishment with most dogs. Reward dovetails with an instinctive canine urge to please. On the other hand, physical punishment frightens most dogs. Fright is counterproductive to training because most dogs will not learn a task when they are frightened. That is particularly the case when housebreaking, because a frightened dog is more apt to panic-soil the floor.

While the vast majority of dogs are successfully housebroken or paper trained, there are a few that never quite get the idea. This generally is the owner's fault, the result of inconsistent training. For example, if a dog intermittently gets away with soiling the floor or carpeting because past mistakes are not discovered for months, then the dog likely will repeat the activity. Products are available at pet stores or through mail order catalogs that deodorize spots where the pet has previously soiled, thus discouraging the pup from returning to the same spot. Once a dog has become an adult and insists on soiling the house, it may be too late for "behavior modification" and the owner must keep the dog confined.

CHEWING

A most annoying and costly devilment is the chewing of shoes, clothing, furniture, or rugs. This occurs in young dogs because they are playful and teething; it occurs in older dogs because they are bored or may resent the owner's absence.

One of the first steps is to get the puppy a chew toy. This may take some experimenting, but after a while a favorite item can be found. Do not give a puppy a piece of personal apparel such as a shoe or slipper to chew on. This sends a mixed signal to an animal that does not have the ability to know the difference between that old throwaway slipper and the nice new leather ones in the closet.

Some dogs will display so-called destructive tendencies to get attention from an owner. At first, this would seem to require more thought processes than dogs possess, but most experts agree that dogs have the mental ability to know what gets them attention and what does not. In some canine minds, negative attention from the owner is better than none at all.

A solution to this problem requires patience and attention to the dog on the owner's part. Simply set aside a few minutes in the morning and evening for time with the dog. Do not inadvertently reward the misbehaving dog by playing with it to divert it after it has begun chewing or some other misbehavior. Instead, voice a sharp "No" and take the item from the dog. Then ignore the dog for about ten minutes. If it behaves, take the dog aside and play with it or groom it. Be sure to wait long enough so that the dog does not connect misbehaving with gaining attention.

Dogs that are eight weeks old generally are able to grasp some of the basic training principles. Keep lessons short, though, no longer than about ten minutes per day until the dog is twelve weeks or older, when lessons can be doubled in length.

Some dogs misbehave whenever the owner leaves the house. One way to break this is for the owner to purposely leave the house for a few minutes, just three or four at first. Few dogs will get into mischief in that brief time. Then return and praise the dog profusely. Continue this regimen for several weeks, gradually increasing the departure time.

Another successful technique for departing owners is to reward the dog prior to leaving the house. Dogs learn to associate the owner's departure with, for example, the rattling of keys, donning of coats, and grabbing of purses or briefcases. But if the owner pauses just before stepping out the door and gives the dog a reward, the dog may not resort to misbehaving. One owner breaks up chunks of a couple of dog biscuits and leaves them "hidden" around the house for the dog to search and eat. Another gives the dog a favorite chew toy that is reserved just for the owner's absence. Such methods may work for a couple of reasons: the dog associates the owner's departure with a reward, or the dog is preoccupied and forgets about the owner's absence.

Some dogs never stop taking advantage of the owner's absence (or sleeping hours) to jump in the owner's bed or to clamber on the sofa. The easiest solution is to close off those rooms or turn sofa or chair cushions on end. It takes just a second, and the dog soon learns that when the cushions are turned, the furniture is definitely off limits.

AGGRESSIVE BEHAVIOR

Aggressive behavior is sometimes a problem, and even young puppies can give a growl or two if their owner is doing something they don't like. The first step in correcting this is to find the cause. A call to the breeder, to a professional trainer, or to a veterinarian may be in order to establish what steps should be taken to curb such behavior.

How to modify aggressive behavior also depends on the extent to which it is occurring. If the dog is constantly picking fights with other family pets or children, then the situation can be grave and may stem from an inherited trait or from improper handling of the pup when it was very young. If the dog is simply testing—snapping or growling at having its toenails clipped, for instance—then a simple, stern "No" may be all that is necessary while the nail clipping task is completed. In some cases, children may be teasing the dog when adults are not around. But if the dog continues or increases its unwarranted attempts to dominate family members or other pets, it probably is best to seek professional advice. Otherwise, the dog may have to be given up. Some aggressive behavior is "treated" by ignoring it and avoiding anything that prompts it, while other nastiness will be made worse if the owner backs down and thus reinforces the behavior. That is why it is crucial to have an accurate assessment of why the dog is behaving aggressively.

TRAINING TIPS

Several ingredients are required for effective dog training. One is to always use the same verbal command for each desired behavior. Another is to strive to use the same neutral tone of voice for commands. Commands given in an overly stern manner may frighten the dog. Keep the praising voice tone more enthusiastic than the commanding tone, with the scolding voice in yet a third tone.

It doesn't matter, really, what the command words are, because the dog responds to voice tone. But it is best to select one-syllable command words and to precede all commands with the dog's name. A food reward is considered the ultimate by most dogs. And keep in mind that intermittent reward actually reinforces training faster than constant reward because it keeps the dog on its toes, striving for the treat.

A final tip: Keep training sessions short. Frequent, short training sessions of about twenty minutes in the beginning for adult dogs, and a maximum of ten minutes for puppies, will achieve the fastest results because short sessions prevent boredom from seeping in and distracting the dog's attention. Ultimately, the adult dog can grow accustomed to work sessions that last about an hour. Stopping work does not hurt the training process. In fact, it seems to help because dogs seem to spend some of their leisure time absorbing the work just completed.

Owners should consider carefully whether to obedience train a dog "formally" or "casually." The formal route is for owners intending to show their dogs. In those cases, owners should teach the basic commands in accordance with show style, that is, proper tension on the lead, the lead in the correct hand, the dog stopping in the correct show stance and exhibiting the proper ring deportment for the breed. Classes are essential for properly educating the handler and the dog for ring work.

Casual training, on the other hand, can be done by any dog owner. Much of the work can be done on the lead or, more informally, off the lead by handling the dog for a few minutes after it has eaten or any time that is convenient and the dog seems willing.

BASIC OBEDIENCE COMMANDS

Every dog, no matter how small the breed, benefits from some basic obedience training. Having a dog that obeys simply makes living with the pet a more pleasant experience. Such training need not take any great time. All that is necessary is a bit of patience and a goal. Most handlers agree that "Come," "Sit," "Stay," "Heel," and "Down" are among the most helpful commands a dog learns.

Teaching a dog the "Come" command is usually first. This can be done any time after age two months, and most dogs catch on especially fast if the owner seizes those opportunities when the dog has chosen to come to the owner. As the dog nears, the owner should repeat "Come," preceded by the dog's name. Once the dog arrives (some take a while), reward profusely. If this is done several times a day, most dogs correctly respond in about a week. Enthusiastic petting

A recommended pet-stain removal method is to take one tablespoon of liquid dishwashing detergent and mix with a half cup of warm water. Dab the stain with a rag and dry with a paper towel. A half-and-half solution of vinegar and water can help remove stubborn stains and accompanying odors.

and voice praising interspersed with food treats will guarantee a dog that wants to come to its owner when called. Young dogs occasionally will playfully duck away just before reaching the owner. Avoid scolding. Just wait the pup out and save the praise for the proper response.

When the dog regularly obeys the "Come" command, proceed to "Sit." Using one hand, gently push the dog's hindquarters into a sitting position while issuing the command. Many puppies will try to play, but just wait the silliness out. Gradually, it will take only a touch to cue the dog to sit down. In a few days, just the command will suffice.

Some owners like to combine the "Come" and "Sit" commands so that the dog will learn to sit as soon as it arrives at the owner's side. It is convenient, but not essential. In fact, it can be more useful to ensure that the dog keeps the two commands separate rather than getting into the habit of automatically sitting every time it arrives after being called.

The owner can choose, of course, in what order to teach the various commands. After "Come," for example, some trainers prefer to teach a dog to "Sit," "Lie down" (or "Down"), and "Stay," in that order. Yet other trainers will teach the dog "Sit," "Stay," and then "Down." The first sequence ("Sit" and then "Lie down") sometimes encourages dogs to habitually lie down immediately after sitting without waiting for the "Lie down" command, which can create a minor problem. But again, it's the owner's decision which sequence of orders to teach.

Teaching the dog to "Stay" can be somewhat taxing on pup and owner and requires extra patience. Invariably the dog is anxious to get to the owner and receive its reward for coming. Once the pup is sitting nicely, the owner should move away while issuing the order "Stay" preceded by the dog's name. At first, the owner will be able to move only a short distance before the dog moves. At that point, command the dog to "Sit" again, and move away again using the "Stay" command. It will take several days of short training sessions before this lessons clicks in the dog's brain. So be patient and do not tackle teaching another command until the dog fully understands the concept of "Stay."

Teaching the dog "Down" usually is not difficult. Most dogs will at first try to pop up out of the down position. When that happens, just apply gentle pressure to the hindquarters and shoulder area to encourage a down position. In some cases, the dog's front feet may have to be moved from their support position. Be sure and praise the dog once it is down, and keep repeating the word "Down" to make the connection between the word signal and the dog's physical position.

Leash-breaking must be done before the pup can be taught to "Heel." Having already taught the dog to "Come" helps with teaching to walk on a lead. Snap the leash on the collar and casually walk along with the dog (dog's choice where, at first) and offer encouragement— "Good dog." Try to keep tension off the lead by speeding up or slowing down to keep up with the dog. This is important, because when a pup first feels tension on a leash, confusion can take over. The dog may sit, lie down, roll over, jump up in the air, and generally fight the lead. Wait out these rough moments. The dog will get up, and when it does, encourage it to "Come" for a reward. Try walking again, and whenever the dog walks nicely on the lead—for even a split second—bend over and give praise or a food reward. Whenever the dog becomes confused or frustrated, fall back on a familiar command so that praise can be given. It is always a good idea to stop a training session on a positive note.

Once the dog understands how to walk nicely on the leash, begin the "Heel" command. When the dog runs ahead or lags behind, give a sharp pull to place the dog next to your left heel and keep offering the command "Heel." As harsh as it sounds, most dogs learn to heel quickly. It is a good command for a dog to know because it makes the daily walks a pleasant experience.

These basic commands are sufficient for the average house pet. Generally, once the dog owner gets the training bug, other commands such as "Fetch" or "Retrieve" are taught. More advanced training includes teaching the dog to jump hurdles and to retrieve after clearing obstacles.

It should be remembered that all dogs are different. Even among the same breeds, some individuals will catch on before others. Owners sometimes grow frustrated with a new puppy that is taking longer than a previously owned dog to learn a task. Just be patient.

SHOWING

Dog shows are held everywhere every year, with the larger shows such as New York's Westminster Kennel Club exhibiting thousands of dogs. In the United States, the official ruling body of dog shows is the American Kennel Club, whose rules govern judging standards at the larger shows.

Dogs entered in breed shows are judged according to the established standards for that particular breed. Even tiny conformation or color flaws can deem an individual dog as "pet-quality" rather than "show-quality." It is wise for the prospective purchaser of a show-quality dog to become educated on the required standards of the breed. Attend shows and talk to breeders and professional show handlers. Reading about the breeds and seeing even the best color photographs cannot substitute for seeing the different breeds in action. Indeed, show judges eye the way a dog moves in order to make their champion selections. Nevertheless, in these classes a judge's subjectivity does come into play.

Somewhat more objective are obedience trials, which can be offered under the auspices of a large show or held as separate events. Breed standards are not important in obedience trials. Dogs must be registered, purebred animals, but they do not have to be perfect breed specimens. Instead, judges score, or rate, the dogs according to the way they obey their handler's bidding. Most obedience trials test dogs in such exercises as heeling, sitting, staying, lying down, standing up, coming when called, retrieving, and tracking scents.

Field trials are another competition available to basset hounds, beagles, dachshunds, the pointing breeds, English springer spaniels, and retrievers. Each performs in a manner suited to that breed: hounds pursue game, pointers point to it, spaniels flush game out, and retrievers fetch it.

To learn how to show a dog properly—that is, once the dog has been deemed appropriate for the show ring—consult local dog clubs, pet stores, or veterinarians to find out when and where classes that teach showing are offered.

66 The one absolutely unselfish friend that a man can have in this selfish world, the one that never deserts him, the one that never proves ungrateful or treacherous, is his dog.
—George Graham Vest 99

CHAPTER **12**

Barks in the Parks

As much as your dog may enjoy new sights and sounds and smells, restrictions on where canines can go in Florida are rather widespread.

FLORIDA'S PARKS

Florida has more than one hundred state parks, including a score of them along lakes and rivers, the Atlantic Ocean, and the Gulf of

Mexico. But some of them are off limits to dogs. The reason, explains the Department of Natural Resources, which is reponsible for the parks, is that dogs can reduce "the quality outdoor recreational experiences" of park visitors. Some parks also feature animals wandering about their natural habitat, and park officials do not want dogs chasing the native creatures. Also of concern to park officials is sanitation, particularly around bathing beaches and concession facilities.

Dogs are not universally barred from state parks. They are permitted in some parks during daylight hours if they are on a six-foot, handheld leash and are well behaved. But unless you know the regulations at a particular park, you may wish to leave your dog at home or back at the hotel.

Not allowed is taking your dog into a state park camping area for an overnight stay. Park officials contend dogs at night can be disturbing to fellow campers. Some campers have suggested that a separate area be maintained in the state parks for pet owners, but the Department of Natural Resources so far has vetoed the idea. It sees developing and maintaining separate areas for dog owners as cost prohibitive.

The foresighted dog owner will call ahead to a state park on his or her itinerary to check pet regulations, even though the visitor has studied that particular park's brochure. There is a good reason to do this. An example is the Stephen Foster Culture Center on the Suwannee River near White Springs. The Stephen Foster park is a vast spread of neatly maintained grass and woods alongside the famous river. It features a museum and a carillion that highlight the music of the nineteenth-century composer. Few wild animals roam the grounds, and therefore park regulations permit dogs on a leash— but only when special events are not being held at the park. Each spring, for example, the park stages a three-day folk festival. At that time, dogs are not permitted in the park, primarily because of the crowds.

The point, then, is not to rely entirely on the policies spelled out in the park brochures. Some are subject to change during special park events. It should also be stated that seeing-eye dogs are exempt from all state park regulations regarding dogs.

Another popular state park that is off limits to Rover is the Ichetucknee River State Park in north Florida, near Fort White. This especially scenic waterway is such a gem of natural Florida flora and fauna that the park also restricts the number of human visitors allowed inside each day and bans motorboats on the pristinely clear waters.

Similar restrictive dog regulations exist in the state's five national forests and the Everglades National Park. Dogs are not allowed on the swimming beaches, in the picnic areas, or on the trails but may be taken into general recreation areas if held on a leash no longer than six feet. Dogs may overnight in the state's national forests and national parks but only if kept confined or leashed.

FLORIDA'S ATTRACTIONS
Unfortunately, your dog also will never get to enjoy Main Street in Walt Disney World's Magic Kingdom or see the killer whales do their

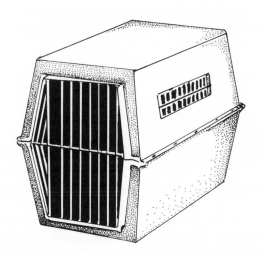

A popular housing choice for small or medium-sized dogs is a plastic shipping crate. These are portable, easy to clean, and can be shut to close in the dog when necessary. They make handy carriers when taking the dog to the veterinarian or for traveling.

> For dog owners who must leave town and do not wish to tote their dog along, an increasing number of in-home pet sitters are available. Before hiring such a sitter, make a thorough check of the service. Ask for references and call prior customers to see if they were happy with the pet sitter.
>
> Once the decision is made to hire an in-home dog sitter, make sure plenty of food and treats are left for the dog to be fed. Sitters report they prefer that the food, can opener, spoons, and medication be left out so that no kitchen rummaging is necessary. Notes should be left informing the sitter of feeding schedules, any special health problems or personality quirks of the pet, and the veterinarian's emergency phone number.

tricks at Sea World. The pet will not get through the gate, even if on a leash or hand carried. Florida's major attractions insist that dogs be kenneled on the grounds—in some cases, at no charge; in other cases, for a fee.

At Sea World, for example, covered kennel cages are stationed in the parking area near the general admission gate. A park visitor puts the dog in one of the cages, shuts the door, locks it, and takes the key. In the cage, the dog has water but no food. After its owner has seen the sights, he or she retrieves the dog on the way back to the car. The kennel service is free.

Walt Disney World, on the other hand, provides a half-dozen kennel areas, including lockups near the Magic Kingdom, EPCOT Center, the studio attraction, and at the Fort Wilderness campground. A visitor to any Disney complex must put the dog in a kennel before passing through the admission gate. There is a daily kennel charge, which includes food and water. No matter how well-behaved your dog, it is not permitted in any of Disney's hotels, either. Overnight guests must kennel them.

FLORIDA'S BEACHES

Florida's primary attraction—its miles of public beaches—also are off limits to dogs, although this policy is often violated and difficult to enforce. The reason for the ban is, of course, sanitation.

Many coastal communities have public beaches maintained by full-time municipal employees that do strictly enforce the ban against dogs meandering among bathers. Enforcement is lax, however, along public waterfront in isolated coastal regions. As a result, a dog retrieving a stick tossed into the surf is a common sight in Florida. Few citations are issued for such frolicking as long as the beach area remains remote and seldom visited by bathers.

TRAVELING TO AND FROM FLORIDA

Considering that so much of Florida's beauty and natural assets, not to mention its famous attractions, are off limits to dogs, one may wonder why a dog wants to come to the Sunshine State. Of course,

To kennel or not to kennel is the dog owner's dilemma at vacation time. Kennel operators report that dog owners sometimes get a little emotional at parting with Bowser, and a dog can become upset, too. Here are a few tips to take some of the worry out of parting with the family pet:

—Take along the pet's favorite toy, rug, or blanket to make the dog feel a little more "at home."

—Check beforehand to see if the kennel owner wants the dog's bed brought along. Some kennel operators say this familiar item goes a long way toward comforting the dog; others say not to bring it because a flea infestation may come along with it.

—Leave good instructions with the kennel. If the dog has peculiarities, such as thunderstorm terrors, tell the kennel personnel.

—Give the kennel a call prior to the drop-off date to see if the dog should be bathed. Some kennel operators prefer the owner bathe the dog before it is brought in for a couple of reasons—to rid the dog of fleas and ticks prior to its boarding, and to keep the dog from having to have a stressful bath at the kennel. Other kennel owners, however, feel just the opposite and like to groom the new arrivals to ensure that they are clean during, or following, their stay.

—Make sure the dog has had its shots so it will not endanger the other boarded dogs with a contagious disease. Similarly, if the dog grows ill prior to the date it is to go the kennel, notify the boarding facility.

—Take along the dog's collar and leash and a supply of your pet's favorite treats.

it's the master's idea, but even he or she may question the move when trying to schedule flying the pet into Florida.

To begin with, air travel can be as traumatic for the owners as for the dog once the owner sees the pet, frightened and perplexed, being stuffed into a crate or cage and placed into a luggage compartment to fly at thirty thousand feet. Nevertheless, airlines and air animal services say that dogs get airborne every day with few catastrophic results.

Flying your dog into or out of Florida requires careful planning. Airline regulations state that dogs cannot board planes up north when the temperature is below 10 degrees, nor can dogs disembark in Florida when the thermometer reads 85 degrees or more at the Florida airport, or at an airport with a Florida connecting flight, such as Atlanta.

Temperatures matter not because the aircraft is too hot or too cold. It is the ground temperature at the airports that is of concern. For example, if temperatures are high in Atlanta, where many Florida flights stop over, the caged dog could be waylaid on a hot tarmac before being loaded aboard the connecting flight to or from Florida. Private animal air services, which use commercial airline service, say they avoid the Florida temperature regulations in the summer months by shipping and receiving dogs during early morning or so-called "red-eye" nighttime flights.

The cost of shipping a dog by air can be expensive. A proper size of airline-approved shipping crate must be purchased, and the flight ticket may exceed a first-class passenger seat. Most large cities have "air-animal" type services that can pick up the dog, ready it for transport, see that it gets on the proper flight, and arrange pickup once the dog has reached its destination.

Shipping a dog by train used to be an alternative, but today's Amtrak does not transport pets of any kind.

A dog wanting to join its master in Florida cannot know the alternative means of getting south, but a considerate owner may best spare the pet potential bad experiences by driving it to its new home. To motor into Florida, a dog need carry only one paper in its suitcase—a health certificate or "clean bill of health" from the family

> Never transport a dog in the bed of an open pickup truck. It is illegal. And veterinarians in Florida treat or euthanize many dogs each year that were injured or maimed because the truck hit a bump and the dog bounced out. At the least, a dog can break its legs, back, or neck if it hits the road hard enough. More serious or fatal injuries occur if the dog falls from the truck into the path of another vehicle. Some dogs also have been dragged or hanged to death because they were connected to the truck by a rope at the time they were thrown from the vehicle.
>
> Humane officials in some Florida counties will issue cruelty citations to persons who carry dogs in the open beds of pickup trucks.

vet. Even then, the owner may not be asked to show it as it crosses into Florida, but the document can be demanded by a stickler who is working one of the numerous agriculture inspection stations guarding the Florida border.

> _**"**I do not know if little dogs cause as large griefs when they die as big ones._
> _—George du Maurier_**"**

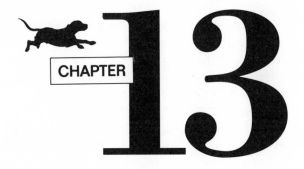

CHAPTER

13

Crossing the Bar

The death of a pet dog can be a particularly difficult time for its owner, especially if the owner is forced to decide whether to have the dog put to sleep. Indeed, deciding to humanely destroy the beloved family dog is undoubtedly the worst aspect of ownership. As a result, say veterinarians, many owners inadvertently permit needless suffering in order to keep their pets alive, even when survival chances are slim and the veterinary bills are rising.

There are some guidelines offered by experts for owners facing this grim decision. One criterion is to assess the dog's overall quality of life. As a dog ages, the owner grows accustomed to a variety of frailties and inconveniences. The dog may be incontinent or suffer loss of sight or hearing. It may become increasingly less mobile and may not eat properly. Still, say some veterinarians, faithful and loving owners rationalize that the dog has a "good life" and "deserves to live." A few owners, especially those who live alone with the animal, actually may feel needed by the increasingly debilitated pet, who in some cases is the only family that the owner has. Aged owners may relate too closely to the aging dog, reasoning that they would not like to be destroyed simply because they have lost their hearing or eyesight.

But dog owners should remember that healthy dogs are naturally active and vital and seek out their owners' attentions. Zest for life is a hallmark of the canine. Once the dog has deteriorated to the point of lying listlessly in a corner, caring little whether it is petted or spoken to, it is time for the owner to question whether the end is, or should be, near.

Just as with human medicine, veterinarians are better able than ever to prolong a dog's life. They specialize in diseases from ophthalmology to orthopedics to cardiology. Diagnostic technology such as ultrasound can better pinpoint a canine disease. But such high-tech equipment can cost a veterinary clinic tens of thousands of dollars to purchase, and specialized equipment and treatment can mean higher bills. Prolonged treatment of some dog ailments can cost an owner thousands of dollars.

Although the average U.S. household spends nearly $100 each year for medical care for the family pet, surveys indicate the dog owner's wallet still is not tapped out. Many dog owners report they would gladly spend more than $500 each year on veterinary care if it meant saving their canine friend.

Spending those dollars is, unfortunately, still no guarantee that the dog's life can be saved. Thus, the pet owner is still faced with the dilemma of determining whether treatment of Fifi or Spot is staying somewhere near the realm of affordability. Even as the veterinary cash register is smoking, an additional humane consideration must be

Lost dogs can be found more easily with new technology. A registration microchip has been developed that can be implanted under a dog's skin in an area between the shoulder blades. The chip is imprinted with an identification code that can be read by personnel at veterinary clinics or humane societies who can call a hot-line number to find the pet's owner.

made: is all the needling, probing, bleeding, X-raying, and confinement in strange surroundings going to improve the dog's quality of life, or is it merely prolonging the dog's life for a mere month or two?

One thing is certain: rare is the veterinarian who will order a dog owner to have the dog put to sleep. As one Florida veterinarian put it, "It is not the role of the veterinarian to make that decision for the owner. That is the owner's decision." Still, veterinarians will offer gentle suggestions, if asked. They can objectively assess whether the dog's future looks bright or not. And the caring owner who takes the time to listen between the lines just may hear the animal doctor saying, "Don't think selfishly of yourself; consider the dog's needs."

A veterinarian with two dogs of his own says, "Knowing that the dog is reaching the end of its life, and caring enough to keep suffering to a minimum, is what truly loving a pet is all about."

WHEN THE END COMES

Behaviorists say that the family dog's death can present as severe a trauma to many folks as the loss of a human companion. In fact, one survey indicated that more than half of the dog owners polled considered their dog as important as any human family member. Indeed, some suicides have been traced to the loss of a pet, particularly if the pet's death occurred in conjunction with other personal problems in the owner's life.

One reason for such acute feelings of loss is simple: true to that old adage, a dog often is man's best friend—at least that is what those who have lost their dogs say. Such adjectives as "irreplaceable" are commonly heard.

Other reasons for profound grief over a pet's death include guilt and the certainty that the lost dog offered the invaluable commodity of unconditional love. "He greeted me when I came home," or "he was always glad to see me," and "my dog listened to me when nobody else would" are the kinds of statements commonly related to veterinarians and friends.

Guilt over the loss of a dog also occurs when the owner believes he or she could have done more to save the animal's life. Thoughts such as "if I had not let the dog stray near the street," or "if only I had noticed that swelling earlier," are, say counselors, part of searching for an explanation for a pet's death.

Yet another form of guilt, say owners whose pets have died, arises from the act of grieving itself. "It's been months now since my dog died, and I still cry over it," said one woman who lost her childhood companion poodle. "And my friends are getting tired of my tears. They cannot understand my feelings and tell me that I should be getting over it and that I should get a new dog. But I feel like getting a new dog is a betrayal to Pierre's memory. I just don't want to go through this again."

Still other bereaved owners frequently point out that "those who have never gone through the grief of losing a pet simply cannot understand what the experience is all about."

More and more counselors are taking grieving pet owners as clients. These counselors as well as veterinarians, who commonly deal with grieving owners, suggest the following measures for coping with the dog's death:

—Strive to treasure the pleasant memories of the pet.
—Don't rush out to replace the lost pet until it sounds like a genuinely good idea.
—Once the decision has been made to find a new dog, consider a breed different from that of the lost pet to avoid grief-evoking comparisons.
—Ignore those who cannot empathize with the grief felt over a lost pet. Be content in the knowledge that grief over a pet's death is a valid emotion even though thoughtless friends or family members may say, "C'mon, it was only a dog."
—Strive to put aside "second-guessing" the attention or treatment given the lost pet. Instead, work at accepting the death as part of the natural cycle of life.

—Do not fib to children about what has happened to the dog. Pet ownership—including loss of the pet—helps children to learn about caring for the dog and dealing with death.

An increasing awareness is developing about the human-animal bond. Hot lines are now available in many major Florida cities to help grieving pet owners express their feelings. Support groups are also available in many locales. They gather to share losses with each other and to hear about lost pets. Owners who feel they need help dealing with their grief can telephone a veterinarian's office for information about hot lines or support groups available in their area.

BURIAL IN FLORIDA

A number of pet cemeteries service pet owners in Florida. They are listed in the Yellow Pages under that category. A surprising number of products such as caskets and headstones are available. Some of the larger pet cemeteries even provide chapels that owners may visit.

Humane societies report that owners who have lost their dogs have a better chance of finding their missing pets if they follow these steps:

1. Start searching for the dog immediately.
2. Pass posters out offering an affordable, but tempting, reward. Keep the posters simple, and if possible, include a good photograph of the dog.
3. Check back regularly with the local humane society or animal shelter to see if the dog has been turned in.
4. Run an ad in the local newspaper's lost-and-found column offering a reward. Supply a general description of the dog, but keep some information secret that allows you alone to make positive identification. Some con artists use the classified lost-and-found notices to bilk money from dog owners.

The more time that passes from the time the dog disappeared, the more unlikely it is that the dog will be returned.

Odds are greater that a missing dog will be returned if it is wearing a collar that bears the owner's name and phone number engraved on a tag. Such tags are available at pet stores, humane society offices, or from mail-order pet suppliers. In most Florida cities, the dog should be wearing a collar that includes its rabies vaccination tag.

Although state law does not forbid burying a pet in the residential back yard, some local laws do prohibit it. If the owner intends to do this, a call to the local health department should be made first. In rural areas, there are few prohibitions against home pet cemeteries, although if the owner lives on rental property the landlord may frown upon the dog's interment.

Another option is cremation. Many pet owners find contentment in having the dog's ashes placed in an attractive urn that can be kept in the home or apartment. One owner says she still enjoys talking to her deceased pet whose remains are kept in a pretty crystal container. "He's still with me," she says.

> **66** *My beagle bit a Kleagle*
> *of the Ku Klux Klan.*
> *—James J. Montague* **99**

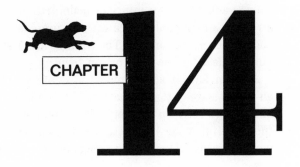

CHAPTER

14

The Legal Beagle

More than a dozen Florida laws mandate the legalities of dog ownership and treatment in the state. Additional local laws exist throughout Florida's sixty-seven counties and hundreds of municipalities. Local ordinances may simply give additional bite to existing state laws or may make their own demands upon persons buying, selling, abandoning, vaccinating, and breeding dogs. Readers are advised to check with the humane societies or animal shelters near them to learn about local laws in their communities.

STATE LAWS REGULATING DOGS AND DOG OWNERSHIP

Abandonment of Dogs

Two state statutes address dog abandonment, which is legally defined as "to forsake entirely or to neglect or refuse to provide or perform the legal obligations of care and support of an animal by its owner or its agent."

Florida statute (FS) 828.13 is an anticruelty law that prohibits leaving a sick, diseased, infirm, or maimed dog to die. It also forbids leaving a dog to suffer injury or malnutrition or dumping a dog off in a street, road, or public place without providing care, food, protection, and shelter for the animal. The offenses are first-degree misdemeanors punishable by a one-year prison term.

Another form of abandonment as defined by FS 705.19 occurs when an owner leaves a dog in the care of a kennel or a licensed veterinarian and fails to retrieve the dog. The kennel or veterinarian must notify the forgetful owner by written notice. The owner then has ten days in which to respond before the kennel or veterinarian may dispose of the dog.

Abandoning a dog that is in the care of a veterinarian also empowers the veterinarian to place a year's lien on the dog owner's personal property for the amount of the unpaid bill (FS 713.655).

Contagious Diseases

It is unlawful, according to FS 828.16, to knowingly sell, trade, or dispose of a dog that has, or has been recently exposed to, a contagious or infectious disease without disclosing that fact to the prospective owner. The statute also prohibits allowing a diseased dog to run loose or to knowingly expose people or other animals to the contagious or infectious dog.

Cruel Confinement

It is against Florida law to keep an animal without giving it sufficient quantities of good quality drinking water and food. Statute

A tourist state, Florida has a large transient population with a small percentage of confidence tricksters who prey on dog owners. One favorite scam takes advantage of owners who have lost their dogs. Law enforcement officials believe the con artists read the local newspaper's lost-and-found column, then call an advertised phone number to report that a lost pet has been found. The owner, often frantic to retrieve the dog, is asked to send money for the dog's safe return. Of course, the dog is never sent home because the con artists never possessed the animal. Some victims of this cruel, money-grubbing hoax report they were threatened by the callers, who said if no money was sent, the lost dog would go to dogfight promoters. Always report such suspicious phone calls to the police or sheriff.

828.13 further forbids keeping any dog in an enclosure without sufficient air or room to exercise.

Cruelty to Animals

This general statute (FS 828.12) provides felony charges against anyone who is cruel to dogs in Florida. Cruel actions include torturing, tormenting, beating, mutilating, or killing. In addition, the statute states that depriving a dog of food or shelter is cruel. Punishment for conviction of the cruelty law is a one-year prison term and a $5,000 fine.

Custody of Neglected or Mistreated Dogs

State law provides that animals deemed to be neglected or abused can be seized by law enforcement officers, agents of the county, or representatives of any society or association for the prevention of cruelty to children or animals (FS 828.073).

Within thirty days of taking the dog into custody, a petition for hearing is filed with a judge in the county where the dog was found. (The statute does not mandate a hearing in the case of stray or abandoned animals.) The hearing must be held within fifteen days after the hearing date is set, and the owner, if known and if residing in the county where the dog was found, must be notified of the hearing within five days after the hearing date is set. If the owner does not live in the county where the dog was seized, notification of the hearing can be published. The purpose of the hearing is to decide whether the owner, if known, can properly take care of the dog in the future. The statute also requires that the seized dog be cared for by county or animal cruelty officials until the court decides whether the animal should or should not be returned to its owner.

If the owner is found by the court to be unable to care properly for the dog, the animal may be auctioned off by the county sheriff. If nobody purchases the dog, it goes back to the county or to animal cruelty officials. The court also may order the dog humanely destroyed. An owner who is found fit to have the dog returned must redeem it within seven days of the court's judgment.

The statute provides several criteria by which county judges determine whether an owner is considered fit. These include:

—testimony from the officials making the seizure as to the condition of the animal and its environment;

—testimony and evidence regarding veterinary care the animal was given after seizure;

—testimony and evidence regarding the type and amount of care the animal received after seizure;

—expert testimony about community standards of proper and reasonable care of similar animals;

—witness testimony regarding prior treatment or condition of this dog or others in the same owner's custody; and

—the past record of the owner and whether there have been prior cruelty convictions.

Burden of proof is on the owner to demonstrate by convincing evidence that he or she is able and fit to have custody of the dog restored and that adequate care will be given the dog in the future.

This statute also provides for the removal of other animals from the owner's premises if he or she is judged to be unfit.

Disposal of Dead Dogs

If buried, a dog's remains must be placed at least two feet below the surface of the ground, according to FS 823.041. The statute warns that it is unlawful to dispose of any animal remains by dumping it on a public road, right of way, or any place where it can be "devoured by beast or bird."

THE LEGAL BEAGLE 159

Dogs for the Disabled

Deaf, blind, visually handicapped, or physically disabled persons have the right granted by FS 413.08 to bring their specially trained dogs into Florida's public accommodations, restaurants, amusement parks, and other places where the general public is invited. In addition, such dogs are permitted onto Florida's common carriers such as airplanes, buses, trains, and other modes of public transportation. The law also stipulates that the dog's owner can be held responsible for any damage done by the dog to any premises or facilities.

Anyone who denies or interferes with a handicapped or impaired person's admittance to or enjoyment of the state's public facilities can be charged with a second-degree misdemeanor punishable by up to sixty days in jail and/or a $500 fine.

Feeding Garbage to a Dog

Florida statute 585.50 prohibits feeding garbage to a dog unless the garbage is heated, cooked, treated, or processed in a way that will render it free of contagious or infectious disease. The law permits an individual to feed household garbage, but only to his or her own dog.

Fighting Dogs

The so-called Animal Fighting Act, FS 828.122, forbids dogfighting as sport. Not only are dog fights illegal, but so is the practice of "baiting," in which a person provokes and harasses a dog into a fighting frenzy for the purpose of training or to promote an actual fight. Baiting is also intended by this statute to include the use of live animals as inducement to racing greyhounds. The statute further prohibits owning, promoting, staging, advertising, managing, operating, or charging admission to any fighting or baiting facility.

Motor Vehicle Accident

Florida statute 768.12 forbids dog owners to take legal action when a collision between an animal and a motor vehicle results in the death of the driver.

Some dog-smart criminals bring along female dogs who are in heat. Male guard dogs thus are sidetracked while the criminal is busy breaking the law.

Poisoning Penalties

Anyone who leaves poisonous substances in any common street, alley, lane, or thoroughfare or in any yard or enclosure other than his or her own can be prosecuted under provision of FS 828.08.

Sterilization of Adopted Dogs

Florida, like all states, is overrun with unwanted dogs. As a result, state law demands that any animals adopted from or purchased from any public or private animal shelter, animal control agency, or humane agency be spayed or neutered. FS 823.15 permits sterilization to be performed prior to turning the animal over to its new owner, or requires that the new owner sign a document promising to have the pet sterilized within thirty days of taking custody or prior to the animal's sexual maturity (around age six months for male and female dogs).

Transporting and Selling Dogs

State law requires any dog brought into Florida to be sold, and any dog purchased in Florida, be inoculated against canine distemper, hepatitis, leptospirosis, tracheobronchitis, and canine parvovirus. The injection must be given no more than thirty days, or less than fourteen days, prior to the dog being brought into Florida. Additionally, a health certificate must accompany each dog sold. For dogs being shipped into Florida from out of state, the certificate must be signed by a veterinarian licensed in the state from which the dog is arriving or by an authorized veterinary inspector of the U.S. Department of Agriculture. The health certificate must show the dog's age, sex, breed, and description, and must include a history of the dog's health as well as the names of the person who is consigning the dog for sale and the person who is accepting the dog for sale. The certificate must also list the vaccines administered to the dog and must state that the animal has no contagious or infectious diseases and is free of intestinal or external parasites, including coccidiosis (an intestinal infection) and ear mites.

Although this statute does not specifically mention rabies, it is an infectious disease, so a dog must be free of rabies to be sold in Florida. Most counties or municipalities in the state require annual rabies shots.

Vicious Dogs

Florida law safeguards people, other domestic pets, and livestock from attack by a biting dog. Several statutes have been enacted that prohibit allowing a dog to commit harm.

One such statute is FS 764.04, which makes the dog's owner liable if a person is bitten while in a public place or lawfully in a private place, including on the dog owner's property. This statute protects any person, such as U.S. mail carriers or utility meter readers. If the victim provoked or aggravated the dog, the owner is not responsible for the victim's injury. Similarly, the dog owner is not liable, the statute says, if at the time the dog bite occurred, an easily read warning sign was posted that contained the words "Bad Dog."

FS 767.01 points out that dog owners are liable for damage done by their dogs to persons, sheep, domestic animals, or livestock. And FS 767.05 assesses liability to the owner of a dog that kills, wounds, or harasses dairy cattle.

In addition to the above laws, still others address the drugging and racing of dogs.

CHAPTER **15**

Canine Camaraderie

The Florida dog can, at its owner's whim, be a social gadabout. Clubs throughout the state cater to breeds and provide shows, obedience trials, and just plain good fun. The following list reveals there's a dog soiree to suit every taste:

FLORIDA DOG CLUBS AND BREED ASSOCIATIONS

Alachua County

Greater Gainesville Dog Fanciers' Assn., Inc.
  Levell Leahy, PO Box 5101, Gainesville, 32602
Marion Alachua Dog Training Assn.
  Janine Tash, Rt. 34, Box 681, Gainesville, 32609

Baker County

Northeast Florida Boxer Club
  Diane Wells, Rt. 2, Box 220, Macclenny, 32063

Bay County

Greater Panama City Dog Fanciers Assn.
  Florence Doty, 7125 Yellow Bluff Rd., Panama City, 32404

Brevard County

Brevard Kennel Club
Tampa Bay Pug Club
  Elizabeth Page, 3965 Richy Rd., Mims, 32754
Central Florida Cairn Terrier Club
  Suzette Heider, 1058 Citrus Ave. NE, Palm Bay, 32905
Indian River Dog Training Club
  Wendy Keighley, 3713 So. Sherwood Circle, Cocoa, 32926

Broward County

Afghan Hound Club of South Florida
  Ed McNamee, 5520 SW 195th Terr., Fort Lauderdale, 33332
Brevard County Dog Training Club
  Patricia Metcalfe, 6975 Glenhaven Ave., Cocoa, 32927
Bulldog Club of South Florida
  Joyce Simmons, 2731 Madison St., Hollywood, 33020
Cocker Spaniel Club of Southeastern Florida, Inc.
  Shere Janzer, 631 No. 65th Ave., Hollywood, 33024
Everglade Golden Retriever Club
  Nancy Carter, 5409 NE 4th Ave., Fort Lauderdale, 33334

Fort Lauderdale Dog Club, Inc.
  Gail Ling, 4741 NW 41st St., Lauderdale Lakes, 33319
German Shepherd Dog Club of Fort Lauderdale
  Angelika Hardesty, 2341 SW 27th Ave., Fort Lauderdale, 33312
Gold Coast Borzoi Club of South Florida
  Rae Petrie-Haas, 2838 Adams St., Hollywood, 33020
Greater Miami Boxer Club
  Donna Budzinski, 4101 NE 4th Ave., Pompano Beach, 33064
Greater Miami Scottish Terrier Club
  Linda Green, 780 SW 75th Terr., Plantation, 33317
Pekingese Club of Southeast Florida
  Nathan Kerr, 605 SW 12th Ave., Fort Lauderdale, 33312
Shetland Sheepdog Club of Greater Miami
  Christine Laughlin, 13411 SW 9th Place, Davie, 33325
Southeast Florida Poodle Club
  Lauren Elardo, 12030 NW 32nd Manor, Sunrise, 33323
Southeast Florida Saluki Club
  Drew Cooney, 2680 NE 12th Ave., Pompano Beach, 33064

Citrus County
Inverness Florida Kennel Club
  Margaret Inman, PO Box 2253, Homosassa Springs, 32647

Collier County
Greater Miami Dog Club, Inc.
  Lois Bradley, 2355 Heritage Trail, Naples, 33962

Dade County
Boston Terrier Club of Miami
  Lucille Sheets, 11601 NW 58th Ave., Hialeah, 33012
Collie Club of Greater Miami
  Felicia Stembach, 11131 SW 69th Terr., Miami, 33173
Dog Obedience Club of Hollywood
  Mary Fielding, 1115 NW 133rd St., North Miami, 33168
German Shepherd Dog Club of Greater Miami
  Barbara Ramos, 12754 SW 46th Lane, Miami, 33175
Miami Obedience Club
  Joanne Bray, 25050 SW 187th Ave., Homestead, 33031

Pembroke Welsh Corgi Club of South Florida
  Cathy DeMott, 20120 NW 15th Ave., Miami, 33169
St. Bernard Club of South Florida
  Charlotte Miller, 1499 West 83rd St., Hialeah, 33014
Shih Tzu Fanciers of Greater Miami
  Betty Blair, PO Box 431469, South Miami, 33243
South Florida Bassett Hound Club
  June Scheiber, 882 NE 146th St., North Miami, 33161
South Florida Miniature Schnauzer Club
  Blanche Glaser, 1719 NE 181st St., North Miami Beach, 33162
Weimaraner Club of South Florida
  Susan Warner, 6630 W. 13th Ct., Hialeah, 33012

Duval County
Afghan Hound Club of Northeast Florida
  Melody Bryan, 681 Chestnut Dr., Jacksonville, 32208
German Shepherd Dog Club of North Florida
  Linda Novotasky, 4183 Ruby Drive E, Jacksonville, 32216
Greater Jacksonville Collie Club
  Patti Merrill, 2040 Sandpiper Point, Neptune Beach, 32233
Greater Orange Park Dog Club, Inc.
  Lani N. Miner, 3324 Lakeshore Blvd., Jacksonville, 32210
Irish Setter Club of Jacksonville
  Sharon Tomore, 1921 Constant Dr., Jacksonville, 32210
Jacksonville Dog Fanciers Assn., Inc.
  Mrs. Diane Heller, 1455 Domas Dr., Jacksonville, 32211
K-9 Obedience Club of Jacksonville
  Betty Jean Shuman, PO Box 52274, Jacksonville, 32201
South Atlantic Cocker Spaniel Club
  Maryrose Picciuolo, 4502 Ortega Farms Circle, Jacksonville, 32210
Sunshine Dachshund Club of Jacksonville
  Mrs. John Hohi, 2633 Loretto Rd., Jacksonville, 32223

Escambia County
Five Flags Dog Training Club of Pensacola
  Angela Cox, 8420 Brickyard Rd., Cantonment, 32533

German Shepherd Dog Club of Pensacola
  Norma Villar, 488 No. 77th Ave., Pensacola, 32506
Pensacola Dog Fanciers Assn., Inc.
  Diana Barron, 5695 Wickford Lane, Pensacola, 32506

Hillsborough County

Bay Area Irish Setter Club of Tampa
  Sharon Carr, 1711 Woodbine, Brandon, 33511
Dog Training Club of Tampa
  Anne Sims, 2610 Watrous Ave., Tampa, 33629
Florida West Coast Doberman Pinscher Club
  Adelaide Combs, 6302 Memorial Hwy., Tampa, 33615
Suncoast Bassett Hound Club of Tampa
  Phyllis Smith, 7310 No. Amos Ave., Tampa, 33614
Tampa Bay Boxer Club
  Jason Zurflieh, Rt. 9, Box 145-B, Tampa, 33610
Tampa Bay Area Shetland Sheepdog Club
  Donna Munsey, 6402 W. Knights-Griffin Rd., Plant City, 33566
Tampa Bay German Shepherd Dog Club
  Brian Porter, 2908 Rogers Ave., Tampa, 33611
Tampa Bay Kennel Club, Inc.
  Genevieve D. Bryant, 2507 Shell Point Rd., Tampa, 33611
Tampa Bay Poodle Club
  Mary Broussard, 609 Green Briar Dr., Brandon, 33511

Lake County

Central Florida Obedience Dog Club
  Ethel Dwyer, Rt 3, Box 813, Eustis, 32726
Lake Eustis Kennel Club
  Denise Stranger-Thorsen, 4455 SR 44, Eustis, 32726
Orlando Dog Training Club
  Patty Blackwelder, 148 W 9th Ave., Mount Dora, 32757

Lee County

Dog Obedience Club of Lee County
  Bonnie Margerum, 2207 River Road SE, Fort Myers, 33905

Fort Myers German Shepherd Dog Club
   Barbara Davis, 6510 Nalie Grande Rd., Fort Myers, 33903
Greater Fort Myers Dog Club
   Mary Jorgensen, 9401 Ligon Court SW, Fort Myers, 33908

Leon County
Tallahassee Dog Obedience Club
   Jill Kuhlman, 1514-C, Dacron Dr., Tallahassee, 32301
Tallahassee Kennel Club
   Virginia Minniear, 530 Collins Dr., Tallahassee, 32303

Marion County
Greater Ocala Dog Club, Inc.
   Lydia Colon, 2109 SW 41st Court, Ocala, 32674

Okaloosa County
Okaloosa Kennel Club, Inc.
   Gina Columbo, PO Box 4621, Fort Walton Beach, 32548

Orange County
Central Florida Kennel Club, Inc.
   Debra Phillips, 915 N. Lakewood Ave., Ocoee, 32761
Keeshond Club of Central Florida
   Linda Cail, 5302 Binnacle Ct., Winter Park, 32792
Orlando Poodle Club
   Joyce Carelli, 4300 McKinnon Rd., Windemere, 32786

Palm Beach County
Boca Raton Dog Club
   Virginia Trout, 196 NE 6th Ave., Delray Beach, 33444
Doberman Pinscher Club of Florida
   Debbie Dyer Pagel, 19575 Liberty Rd., Boca Raton, 33434
Florida East Coast Dachshund Club
   Sandra Bayley, 20897 Hamaca Ct., Boca Raton, 33433
Great Dane Club of South Florida
   Diane Raiford, 7763 Granada Blvd., Miramar, 33023

Jupiter-Tequesta Dog Club, Inc.
    Gail Klein, 23956 Mallard Creek Dr., Palm Beach Gardens, 33418
Obedience Training Club of Palm Beach County
    William Engle, 1040 Forest Ct., West Palm Beach, 33405
Palm Beach County Dog Fanciers Assn.
    Mrs. C. E. Davis, 3700 Joseph Dr., West Palm Beach, 33417

Pasco County
Central Florida Brittany Club
    Lisa Hampton, 7313 University Dr., Hudson, 33567
Pasco Florida Kennel Club
    Martha Ooms, 331 Twenty Mile Level Rd., Land O'Lakes, 34639

Pinellas County
Clearwater Kennel Club
    Judy Rinaldi, 1256 Alhambra Court, Palm Harbor, 34683
Dog Training Club of St. Petersburg
    Desma West, 665 Villa Grande Ave. So., St. Petersburg, 33707
Florida West Coast Miniature Schnauzer
    Joy Hathaway, 2401 Country Trails Dr., Safety Harbor, 34695
St. Petersburg Dog Fanciers Assn., Inc.
    Patricia Tatham, 4834 Lake Charles Dr. No., Kenneth City, 33709
Tampa Bay Bulldog Club
    Carol Flynn, 4501 38th St. So., St. Petersburg, 33711
Upper Suncoast Dog Obedience Club
    Melenie Paul, PO Box 1526, Dunedin, 34296

Polk County
Great Dane Club of Mid-Florida
    Elizabeth Johnson, 1018 Haymarket Dr., Lakeland, 33809
Imperial Polk Obedience Club of Lakeland
    Laura Carew, 1920 East Edgewood Dr., Lakeland, 33803
Lakeland Winter Haven Kennel Club, Inc.
    Jan Brungard, PO Box 1047, Haines City, 33844
Mid-Florida Shetland Sheepdog Club
    Catherine Grafstrom, 2332 York Place, Lakeland, 33809

St. Lucie County
Treasure Coast Kennel Club of Florida, Inc.
   Agnes Siple, 1082 SW Sultan Dr., Port St. Lucie, 33453

Sarasota County
Florida East Coast Dachshund Club
   Mary Castoral, 2705 Norwood Lane, Venice, 33595
Florida Gulf Coast Weimaraner Club
   Barbara Heller, 4436 Westwood Lane, Sarasota, 34231
Greater Venice Florida Dog Club, Inc.
   William Zimmerman, 427 Mexicali Ave., Venice, 33595
Manatee Kennel Club, Inc.
   Barbara M. Mitchell, 2181 Shadow Oaks Rd., Sarasota, 34240
Sara Bay Kennel Club, Inc.
   Paulette Braun, 1500 No. Orange 42, Sarasota, 34236
Sarasota Obedience Training Club
   Ron Carver, 235 Grant Ave., Sarasota, 33579
Tampa Bay Chihuahua Club
   Bette Ann Roupp, 5042 Lahaina Dr., Sarasota, 33582

Seminole County
German Shorthaired Pointer Club of North Florida
   Margaret Seybert, 1983 Ranchland Trail, Longwood, 32750
Seminole Dog Fanciers Assn.
   Lynn Sutay, 1875 Stone St., Oviedo, 32765

Volusia County
Greater Daytona Dog Fanciers' Assn., Inc.
   Janet Stasiak, 357 Collins St., Ormond Beach, 32074
Greater German Shepherd Dog Club of Orlando
   Barbara Stoddard, 494 Western Rd, New Smyrna Beach, 32069
Obedience Club of Daytona
   Jeanette Pearson, 682 Gaslight Dr., South Daytona, 32019
West Volusia Kennel Club
   Nancy Boltz, 135 DeLeon Rd., DeBary, 32713

GLOSSARY

Anal glands Situated on either side of the dog's anus, these glands can become impacted. A signal of impaction is the dog scraping its hindquarters along the grass. Once impaction occurs, the glands must be cleared, a job best done by the veterinarian. Some references indicate that well-exercised dogs suffer fewer impactions.

Balanced A proportioned appearance that indicates all the individual body parts are the proper size. Varies from breed to breed.

Bitch A female dog.

Bite The proper (or improper) position of the teeth when they are closed. A correct bite for the dog is a "scissors" bite in which the lower teeth close cleanly behind the upper teeth.

Bone The overall substance or heft of a dog's appearance.

Breeder As recognized by the American Kennel Club, the owner of the mother of the puppies.

Brindle Usually brown, tan, or gray coloring mixed evenly with black hairs.

Canine teeth The sharp fangs on the upper and lower jaws.

Chops The bulldoglike jowls of a dog.

Cropping The cutting of a dog's ear to make it stand up alertly. Doberman pinschers and Great Danes are two breeds that generally have their ears trimmed sometime between the age of six weeks and four months.

Crossbred A dog with two different breeds of parents.

Cynology The study of canines.

Dam The mother of puppies.

Dewclaw An extra toenail found on the inside of the leg and thought to be the remains of a vestigal fifth toe.

Dewlap A portion of extra skin that hangs under the dog's throat. Seen in loose-skinned breeds such as the bloodhound.

Fall Hair that hangs over the dog's face.

Feathering Fringe of hair on certain areas such as the tail, legs, or ears.

Flews Hanging regions of the upper lips found in breeds such as the Great Dane.

Geld To remove (castrate) the testicles of a male dog. More commonly called *neutering* in the United States.

Guard hairs The longer, stiff hairs that add sheen to the coat and overlie the softer undercoat.

Hackles Bristles of hair on the back and neck that rise when a dog is frightened or aggressive.

Heat Euphemistically known as "in season," the heat cycle indicates when a female dog is ready to be bred. Depending on the breed, this may occur from once to several times each year. The onset of these cycles may occur as early as six months in some breeds and is sure to attract every rogue male dog in the neighborhood. As a word of caution, dogs have been known to breed through chain-link fence.

Inbreeding The breeding of related dogs to one another. Many breeders regularly breed brother and sister dogs to one another, with some swearing that it produces better offspring. Today, the practice occurs less often as more physical and mental defects are identified as hereditary.

Outcross breeding Breeding dogs together who are free from any common ancestry for many generations.

Rough coat A shaggy or longhaired coat.

Sire A puppy's male parent.

Smooth coat Closely lying short hair.

Spay To surgically remove a female dog's reproductive organs.

Weaning The withholding of mother's milk from her puppies. Most pups are weaned at about five weeks old. At about three weeks, pups often will signal growing interest in food other than milk and can be fed small amounts of semisolid food.

Whelping The act of a mother dog giving birth. Generally, nature takes care of the process, but if the dam is having undue difficulty a veterinarian should be summoned. Some owners provide special whelping boxes for the expectant mother. Many dogs will choose their own location unless confined.

Index